Sugar Detox Plan & Fatty Liver Diet

© Copyright 2018 by Charlie Mason - All rights reserved.

The following Book is reproduced below with the goal of providing information that is as accurate and reliable as possible. Regardless, purchasing this Book can be seen as consent to the fact that both the publisher and the author of this book are in no way experts on the topics discussed within and that any recommendations or suggestions that are made herein are for entertainment purposes only. Professionals should be consulted as needed prior to undertaking any of the action endorsed herein.

This declaration is deemed fair and valid by both the American Bar Association and the Committee of Publishers Association and is legally binding throughout the United States.

Furthermore, the transmission, duplication, or reproduction of any of the following work including specific information will be considered an illegal act irrespective of if it is done electronically or in print. This extends to creating a secondary or tertiary copy of the work or a recorded copy and is only allowed with the express written consent from the Publisher. All additional rights reserved.

The information in the following pages is broadly considered a truthful and accurate account of facts and as such, any inattention, use, or misuse of the information in question by the reader will render any resulting actions solely under their purview. There are no scenarios in which the publisher or the original author of this work can be in any fashion deemed liable for any hardship or damages that may befall them after undertaking information described herein.

Additionally, the information in the following pages is intended only for informational purposes and should thus be thought of as universal. As befitting its nature, it is presented without assurance regarding its prolonged validity or interim quality. Trademarks that are mentioned are done without written consent and can in no way be considered an endorsement from the trademark holder.

BONUS:

As promised, please use your link below to claim your 3 FREE Cookbooks on Health, Fitness & Dieting Instantly

tiny.cc/qzu27y

You can also share your link with your friends and families whom you think that can benefit from the cookbooks or you can forward them the link as a gift!

Table of Contents

BONUS: 4
Introduction 12
Chapter 1: The Basics of Detox 14
What Are Toxins? 14
The Benefits of Going on a Detox 15
Different Types of Detox 18
A Cleanse Versus a Detox 20
Chapter 2: How to Get Started on a Detox 22
Take Measurements of Yourself 22
Out with the Bad 23
In with the Good 24
Prepare for the Crash 24
Add In Some Simple Lifestyle Practices 26
Foods to Eat During a Detox 27
Some Things to Consider When You Are on a Detox 28
Chapter 3: Simple Steps to Reduce Inflammation in the Body 30
Get Some Omega-3 Fatty Acids in Your Diet 30
Eat Some Herbs 31
Be Careful About the Types of Fats You Consume 32
Refined Carbs and Sugars Are the Enemies 33
Eat Foods That Are Rich in Antioxidants 34
Take Some More Vitamin D in Your Diet 35
What Do These All Have in Common? 35
Chapter 4: Improving Your Immune System Through a Detox 38
Foods That Clean Out the Body 39

The Best Foods for Boosting Your Immune System............41
Your Ultimate Nutrition and Vitamins Plan 42
    Vitamin C 43
    Vitamin E 44
    Vitamin A 44
    Vitamin D 44
    Folate or folic acid 45
    Iron 45
    Selenium...46
    Zinc 46

Chapter 5: Ending Your Sugar and Carb Cravings 47
Why Are We Addicted to Sugar? 48
How to Go on a Sugar Detox 51
Tips to Make a Sugar Detox Easier 55

Chapter 6: Easy Habits That You Can Adopt to Kick Those Sugar Cravings Out 58
Replace Your Evening Snack with a Fruit 58
Plan Out Your Meals Ahead of Time 59
Clean Out the Kitchen to Avoid Temptations 59
Drink Some Water When You Have a Craving 60
Eat Healthy Meals 60
Identify Your Triggers 61
Take In Enough Complex Carbs 62

Conclusion 64

Fatty Liver Diet: 66

Introduction 67
A Few Things to Know About the Safety of Liver Detoxes .68
Keep Your Liver Healthy 69

The Main Reasons for Completing a Liver Detox for Preventing and Curing Fatty Liver Disease 70

Chapter 1: What Is Fatty Liver Disease? 73
Alcohol-Related Fatty Liver Disease or ALD 73
Non-Alcoholic Fatty Liver Disease or NAFLD 77
    Risk Factors 79
        Liver Cancer 80

Chapter 2: How the Liver Functions and Types of Liver Disease 83
What Are the Different Types of Liver Disease? 85
    Viral Infections 86
    Parasitic Liver Infections 86
    Alcoholic Liver Disease 86
    Autoimmune Repercussions 87
    Genetic Disorders 87
    Growths, Tumors, and Cancer 87
    Cirrhosis 88
    Pediatric Liver Conditions 88
Signals of Liver Issues 89
    Jaundice or Yellowed Eyes and Skin 89
    Dark Urine And/Or Pale Stool 89
    Pain in the Liver 89
    Easy to Bruise 90
    Additional Signals to Watch out For: 90
Liver Disease Diagnosis 90

Chapter 3: What Is a Liver Detox? 92
The Most Common Liver Detoxes 92
Common Detox Symptoms 94
The Best Detox Solution for You 95

Chapter 4: The Benefits of a Liver Detox 97

Chapter 5: How to Detox Your Liver Through Diet... 99

Tip 1: Eliminate or Minimize Foods That Are Toxic to Your Body 99

Tip #2: Juice Made from Raw Vegetables Is an Effective Delivery Method of Nutrients 100

Tip #3: Foods Rich in Potassium Are Essential 101

    Sweet Potato 102

    Tomato Sauce 102

    Leafy Greens 103

    Beans 104

    Molasses 104

    Banana 104

Tip #4: Do an Enema with Coffee 105

Tip #5: Supplements for Turmeric, Dandelion, and Milk Thistle Are Beneficial 106

    Turmeric 106

    Dandelion 106

    Milk Thistle 106

    Bonus! Burdock Root 107

Tip #6: Take Liver Supplements or Eat Organic Liver Meat Regularly 107

Chapter 6: Natural Remedies for Fatty Liver Disease 108

Current Natural Remedy Findings for Treating NAFLD ..109

    Goji Berry, Wolfberry, or Lycii Fructus 109

    Garlic or Allium Sativum 109

    Green Tea 110

    Resveratrol 110

Milk Thistle 111

Additional Decoctions and Derivatives to Consider 111

Additional Natural Suggestions 112

Chapter 7: Healthy Diet Foods and Drinks for Fatty Liver Disease 113

How to Heal Fatty Liver Disease Through Food 114

Additional Liver-Supporting Foods 117

Additional Liver-Supporting Beverages 118

Avoid the Following Foods: 119

An Example Diet Plan 120

Additional Natural Remedies Suggestions for Fatty Liver Disease 121

Chapter 8: Eating Plans and What Foods and Drinks to Avoid 123

Foods to Avoid in Your Liver Detox Eating Plan 124

Tips on How to Get the Most from Your Liver Detox Eating Plan 124

Eating Plan Menu and Detox Plan Sample 126

Friday Evening 126

Saturday Early Morning 126

Saturday Late Morning 126

Saturday Afternoon 127

Saturday Late Afternoon 127

Saturday Night 127

Sunday Early Morning 127

Sunday Afternoon 128

Sunday Late Afternoon 128

Sunday Night 128

Monday Morning Through Night 128

A 24-Hour Liver Detox 129

24-Hour Detox Drink 129
Easy Detox Soup Recipes 130
   Broccoli Soup..130
   Beet Soup 131
Conclusion **133**

Sugar Detox

Guide to End Sugar Cravings (Carb Carving)

Introduction

Congratulations on purchasing the *Sugar Detox*, and thank you for doing so.

When you hear the word detox, you may automatically assume that this means you will spend weeks on a diet plan that contains hardly any calories—maybe even drinking most of your nutrition, in the hopes of cleaning out the body and losing weight. While there are detoxes that are like this, there are other ones that are more about reducing harmful chemicals and food sources from your diet so that you can clean out the body and feel healthier and more energized in no time. That is how the sugar detox works.

Sugar is all around us. We can't go into the grocery store without a million signs about the newest baked good that is out there. We see it in commercials, find it in our snacks, and even discover it hidden in our canned goods. It is even hidden in some of the foods that we usually consider healthy.

What makes it worse is that there are also a ton of refined carbs that can be just as bad. These are the white bread, white pasta, and white flours that make up many baked goods. These may be listed differently on the label, but once the body absorbs them, they are converted over into more sugars, making the problem even worse.

Eating too much sugar in your diet can cause a whole host of health problems. It can make you feel sick, ruin your immune system, add on the pounds, and even add more inflammation to the body. Additionally, the more sugar that you eat, the worse the problem is going to get. This becomes a vicious cycle of always craving more sugar and not being able to get enough. Getting out of this cycle can be really hard to accomplish.

A sugar detox aims to help break this cycle. It helps you eliminate the sugars that you consume, even taking out fruits in some cases, to help you get in better health. There may be a crash, and there is going to be some tough times, but going through this sugar detox will be one of the best things that you can do for your overall health.

This guidebook is going to spend some time talking about how to get started with a sugar detox, some of the steps that you need to follow, the importance of eating the right foods to help with building up your immune system and fighting off inflammation, and some of the things you can do to help stay on a sugar detox for the long term.

No matter what health condition you are dealing with, or if you just want to finally get over a sugar addiction that has been bothering you for some time, going on a sugar detox is the best way to help you out. This guidebook will give you the advice and tips that you need to get started.

There are plenty of books on this subject on the market—thanks again for choosing this one! Every effort was made to ensure it is full of as much useful information as possible. Please enjoy!

Chapter 1: The Basics of Detox

To keep things simple, a detox is a process that a person takes in order to make various lifestyle changes to help clear their body of the toxins that are inside. Sometimes, you will detox to get ready for an intense diet plan, and other times, you just want to create more mental clarity and energy in the body. These lifestyle changes would often include abstaining from certain things that are considered harmful to help optimize the processes of the body. Some of these changes are going to be temporary, while others are going to be more permanent.

What Are Toxins?

Before we move on, it is important to discuss toxins and what they mean before you go on a detox. Toxins are any substance that is considered poisonous or that could cause negative health effects because of their presence. Toxins can refer to artificial food ingredients, pollutants, chemicals, metals, pesticides, poisons, and even sugars that could cause some harm to the body.

Toxin is a very broad term and there are many things that can be included under it. Remember that we are in constant contact with pollutants and harmful organisms. These show up in our air, our food, and our water—and it is virtually impossible to get away from them. Oftentimes, the toxins that we are trying to clear out in our bodies are the ones that build up over years.

There isn't much you can do to help protect the body from the toxins that are found in the environment. However, there are ways to get rid of the toxins that come from the foods that you eat. A detox helps you change up some parts of your lifestyle so that you can clear out the body and stay as healthy as possible.

In some cases, the body is able to detox itself, if you give it the time. For example, some people will choose to go on a sugar-free diet. They will abstain from sugar as much as possible. During that time, the body will work to eliminate the extra sugar that is there and repair the damage. Sometimes you have to give the body some time to do the work, but by simply removing the toxin from your life, you can see improvements.

A detox can help you reduce these toxins from the body. By eating the right foods and ensuring that you make some changes in your diet, you are going to see some amazing results. The toxins will leave the body, you will have more energy, and some health conditions will fix themselves with just a few weeks on the right detox plan.

The Benefits of Going on a Detox

At this point, you may wonder why you would choose to go on a detox plan, to begin with. Aren't these just fads—things that aren't going to last at all and will make you feel worn out and with no real results long term? There are actually a lot of benefits of going on a detox, and it is something that everyone should consider. Some of the best benefits of choosing a detox plan include the following:

- Gives your body more energy: When you flush those toxins out of the body, you will feel more lively and energetic. While you detox, you are also stopping the influx of saturated fats, trans fat, caffeine, and sugar—and then replacing them with more natural foods, like fruits and vegetables. You can enjoy that natural energy burst without any of the crash that normally comes.

- Gets rid of the extra waste: The biggest reason people go on a detox is to allow the body some time to get rid of any extra waste it is storing. These programs are meant to stimulate the body to clean itself out, including the colons, kidneys, and liver. Most diseases that you are at risk for will be caused by storing waste in the body, which is why this detoxification is so important.

- Helps you with weight loss: Yes, with the detox you are only going to lose weight for the short term. You will have to maintain a healthy lifestyle and eating habits to see the weight loss tick around, but that is true of any type of plan. If you look at this detox program as a method that can establish long-term eating habits and as a way to get rid of habits that are unhealthy, then it is a good thing. If you only go on the detox as a way to get rapid weight loss, then you will gain the weight back.

- Stronger immune system: Those who choose to go on a detox are going to see that their immune system is stronger. When you clear out some of the bad stuff, the stomach is better able to handle the nutrients that you take in, including Vitamin C. A good detox program is going to have some recommended intake of herbs that can help the lymphatic system. This is an important player in ensuring you stay healthy for the long term.

- Improved skin: Your skin is a huge organ, the large one you have. Since a good detox program is able to improve your overall health, it makes sense that the skin is going to benefit the most.

- Better breath: Some people state that going on a detox is a good way to help them get a better breath. If you have been suffering from issues of bad breath, and nothing seems to be working, then it may be time to try out a detox and see what it can do for you.
- Promotes some healthy changes: The amount of time that you are on a detox may vary, but the changes it can make to your lifestyle are really long-term. If you use it properly, this detox can be a gateway to your life being healthier.
- Clearer thinking: Not only does the detox help out your body, but it can strengthen your mind. With all those toxins gone and replaced with healthier nutrients, the brain is able to function in a way you had forgotten was possible.
- Healthier hair: All the herbs, minerals, and vitamins that you will take in during the detox can really help make your hair shine like never before.
- Feeling lighter: Many people state that when they go on a detox, they start to feel lighter. All that sugar and fat can make your body feel weighed down, but when you kick it out through a detox, you are going to naturally feel lighter.

Different Types of Detox

You may be surprised at all the different types of detoxes that are out there. You can go on a detox for almost anything that you want, depending on which part of your body you want to improve or what toxin you want to get rid of. Some of the different options that you can choose for a detox include:

- Colon Cleanse: While the colon has an important job to do, sometimes it may need a bit of help get the job done. Sometimes you will use water, fiber, and a supplement to help out.

- Liver Cleanse: Many times the liver cleanse is going to be done by eating certain types of foods or taking a supplement. However, if you do use a supplement that is supposed to help out with this, you should be careful. Some studies show that these supplements don't really work how they advertise and that they could end up causing harm to the body.

- The Master Cleanse: This is an idea that has been around for some time, but many celebrities are making it popular now. To do this kind of cleanse, you are going to drink a concoction of cayenne pepper, maple syrup, and lemon water. You would then have it along with an herbal detox tea. Do this daily for a minimum of ten days, and have nothing else. It does work short term to help you lose weight, but it is not a fun detox and can make you cranky and irritable.

- The Green Smoothie Cleanse: Pictures of green smoothies seem to pop up every once in a while as people decide it is time to try out one of these cleanses. Depending on how they go, some participants are able to drop up to 15 pounds simply by drinking smoothies that are made out of veggies and fruits. They do this for ten days. This could cause problems because you are missing out on nutrients like protein, but doing it for a day or two to restart the system may be fine.

- Juice Cleanse: This is a good way to help you get lots of minerals and vitamins out of your produce, without having to sit there and chew on them all day long. There are a lot of these cleanses, but they have the advantage of really overdosing you with lots of vitamins and minerals. These often contain a lot of sugar, unless you really emphasize the vegetables and leave most of the fruits out.

- Detox Cleanse: Detoxing, or the process of taking unhealthy toxins out of the body, is one of the main reasons that people will go on a cleanse. Toxic overload can make you feel sluggish, can lead to a lot of acne, and can cause many allergic reactions. Going on a detox can help the body naturally get rid of the toxins and feel better.

- Dherbs Full-Body Cleanse: Dherbs is a company that makes a line of proprietary supplements that are meant to help with a range of health problems and illnesses. The full-body cleanse will give you liquid supplements or pills that you use each day for 20 days, and you use a raw food diet they suggest. This can be a way to lose a lot of weight, but information on it is pretty slim. Hence, it is best to go cautiously with it.

- The Sugar Detox: Many people consume way too many carbs and sugars in their day. When the sugar isn't being used up by the body, it is going to stick around and cause problems to the organs, diabetes, heart conditions, and more. A sugar detox aims to reduce the refined carbs and the sugars from the diet and replace them with healthier meal alternatives.

These are just a few of the detox options that you can choose to go with. They are all meant to help clean out the body and make you feel more energized and prevent a ton of health conditions all at the same time.

A Cleanse Versus a Detox

When you are looking for methods to help improve your health or to help you lose weight quickly, two words that you are going to hear often include cleanse and detox. Many people assume that these two are the same thing, but there are some differences.

You can use both of them to help clean out the body and help you lose weight. But there are some key differences that come with a detox diet and a cleanse. First, let's look at a detox. Assuming that you don't fall into a radioactive swamp someday, your body is actually equipped to help you deal with most of the toxins it encounters. When you inhale, absorb, or ingest toxins—the kidneys and the liver are going to work to help flush these toxins out. This is something that the body has been doing long before detoxes and cleanses were important.

However, if you end up hammering your body with common environmental toxins and skimping on proper hydration and nutrients, the natural detoxification system of the body will be in trouble. Your body wants to naturally get rid of all those toxins and other unhealthy things. But then, if you keep eating lots of junk, it is hard to get the original junk out at all. You are basically just clogging the drain in this situation. Over time, if you don't fix this issue, it can put your kidneys and liver under a lot of pressure, and this is where the process of cleansing comes into play.

To help the body get back to its natural detoxing process, you are going to need to eliminate some of the toxins. One of the best ways to do this is to reduce or eliminate some of the junk that you usually eat and to replace that with an abundance of healthy foods. This helps flood the body with lots of nutrients that can help the body get its job done faster.

There are many different detoxes available, including the ones that we discussed above—but the point is to help you stop taking in some of the different toxins, such as alcohol, sugars, and refined carbs from your diet. They also focus on eating lots of healthy foods, especially fresh fruits and vegetables, so the body has enough nutrients to finish flushing out the bad stuff.

Chapter 2: How to Get Started on a Detox

Getting started with a detox does not have to be difficult. In fact, the more natural you make it, without completely shocking your system (at least for more than a few days), the easier it will be on your body. Having a plan in place can often make the whole process easier. Let's look at some of the steps that you can follow, no matter what kind of detox you decide to go on.

Take Measurements of Yourself

Before you start on the detox program, do some measurements. It is fine to take your weight, but there are also other things that you want to measure to help you see how effective the detox can be. You can record these answers in a notebook of your choice or record them on your computer to help you get a good starting point.

Start by weighing yourself. Do this right away in the morning, when you have had time to fast because you were asleep. Do this without clothes on and after you go to the bathroom to get the best results. You can then measure your hips and your waistline. Using a tape measure, find the widest point around the belly button to get the waist.

You can choose if you want to measure out anything else. Some people include this detox with a new exercise program, and they want to see the results of that as well. They may measure bust size, arms, legs, and more to help them see the results.
Then, when the detox is done—or at regular intervals—if this detox is going to become a more permanent part of your lifestyle (which is often what happens with a sugar detox), make sure to take mea-

surements again. This helps you see your progress and see how great this detox can be.

Out with the Bad

When you are ready to start on a detox, it is time to get rid of all the bad that is in your diet. Get rid of the junk food that is hiding in your fridge and cabinets. Anything that contains toxic ingredients, especially sugar, should be set aside or tossed out. During the detox, and hopefully longer once you get used to it, you will not eat anything that has added sugars or is processed. Some of the things that you need to toss out, or at least keep to the side, include:

- Anything that wouldn't be considered real food, i.e. anything that comes in a package, box, or a can. Options like whole foods that are found in a can, such as artichokes with water or sardines, may be fine.
- Any drink or food that has any added sugar. This includes options like artificial sweeteners, organic cane juice, agave, molasses, maple syrup, and honey.

- Anything that contains refined vegetable oils or hydrogenated oils.

- Any foods that have dyes, coloring, additives, preservatives, and artificial sweeteners. Anything that has been processed should be eliminated.

- Alcohol: Many alcohols have a lot of sugars in them, so make sure to avoid them when you go with a detox.

- Dairy products: While dairy products can be good for you, during this time, you should avoid them. They often contain high amounts of sugar that can be hard on the body and can induce cravings. After the initial part of the detox, you can decide to add it back in, sparingly, if you would like.

In with the Good

For the remainder of your detox, many of which are ten days long, you are going to focus on flooding your body with the nutrients that it needs. These nutrients are going to help the body repair itself in a more natural way, getting rid of that sugar, and helping you look and feel your very best. After the first few days, your body will feel so energized and renewed, that you won't even want to eat the sugars any longer.

During this phase, you may want to set up some meal plans. Those sugar and carb cravings are going to be tough. Having a plan in place can really make a difference and help you stay on track. Plan for all your meals, along with some snacks, so you don't even need to think about what you are eating—it is all prepared and ready for you.

Prepare for the Crash

If you are going on a sugar detox, be prepared for the hard crash when you first start. Our bodies crave sugar, even though it is bad for us. In our past, many people had to rely on sugar to help them out. This sugar was a great source of energy when there was famine or longer periods without eating. Finding something sweet to eat and getting as much of it as possible was a way to help keep people alive.

Unfortunately, that same idea is still prevalent in our systems today. And in a modern world where sugar is always available, this is not necessarily a good thing. We no longer need sugar to survive. There is no risk of famine in most of the western world, which means that the role of sugar is not that important any longer.

Despite this, those cravings for sugar are very strong. It is hard to get rid of them. Even if we eat a lot of it during the day, we are going to crave some more by the end of the day. We know that eating too much is bad, but we also find that it is very hard to stop—and we just keep eating it over and over again. This, over time, causes health conditions like heart disease, stroke, and diabetes.

When you decide to go on a sugar detox, you are effectively taking the steady stream of sugar out of your life and trying to replace it with something healthier. However, the body is going to revolt. That energy high you got from the sugar is going to be gone, and those cravings are going to kick in hard. You are going to be tired, grumpy, and you will want some sugar right then and there. But you have to remain strong. After a few days, you will start to feel better—without the sugar crash—and you will see just why cutting out sugar is the best.

If you have a really strong addiction to sugar, this process may be harder. Some people like this decide to completely get rid of sugars, at least as much as they can. They will go on a detox that completely gets rid of fruits and even some whole grains. While the sugars in these are healthy and considered good for the body, sometimes, it is best to drop them for a few weeks so that you can get over that sugar addiction faster. Later, when your body has had time to adapt, you can add them back into the diet slowly without having to worry about your hard work going down the drain.

Therefore, no matter which type of fast you choose to go on, you need to be prepared for a crash. Have some good meals put in the freezer—ones that will give your body the nutrients it needs to make it through this process. It only lasts a few days, so it isn't too bad. However, some people find this is the hardest part of the whole detox process.

Add In Some Simple Lifestyle Practices

While changing out your diet can be an important part of a detox, there are a few other things that you need to focus on as well. Changing up some of your lifestyle habits can make a big difference in how well the detox works and how good you feel when it is done. Some of the things that you can add into your lifestyle to make the detox more effective include:

- Get enough sleep—seven to eight hours a night is the best.
- Spend five minutes doing some deep breathing.
- Drink at least 8 glasses of water each day.
- Spend 15 minutes journaling about your day.
- Be active during the day. Get up and do a walk or some other physical activity for a minimum of 30 minutes a day.
- Take fiber before every meal to help balance your blood sugars, and cut out cravings.
- Take a good multivitamin.
- Take a detox bath. A good one to go with is 2 cups of Epsom salt, 10 drops of lavender oil, and ½ cup of baking soda.

Add these steps to following the specific rules of a detox, and you are going to find that going on a detox can actually be pretty easy. You may have to deal with some of the cravings for the first few days. Nevertheless, as the body cleans itself out some more, you will find that it is a great way to make you feel good and to get your health up and running again.

Foods to Eat During a Detox

Eating on a detox is not meant to be difficult. You simply need to cut out some of the junk in your diet and focus more on the healthy foods rather than the junk found in a traditional American diet. First, you need to focus on eating lots of healthy fruits and vegetables. All produce can be great for a detox. Just try to get a large variety so you that can get all the nutrients your body needs.

Next, focus on whole grains. These whole grains are going to help fill you up, balance your blood sugar levels, and contain a lot of great nutrients as well. Make sure that you stick with whole grain options rather than refined grains. The refined grains turn into sugars in the body and can make a sugar detox almost impossible. Meanwhile, whole grains provide your body with everything that it needs, without any of the bad stuff.

Lean meats are important as well, especially fish. Fish provides you with all of the nutrients you need, with none of the bad fats that can cause inflammation and harm your health. You can choose other meats as well. Lean poultry products are good as well. It is best to stick away from some options like bacon and beef, other than having it occasionally.

When you first get started on a sugar detox, it is best to hold off on the milk products. These products have a lot of extra sugars inside them, which can make them a bad decision to add in when you want to get rid of sugar. They also contain higher amounts of carbs, and they can be a dangerous thing, especially on this kind of detox. Stick with other options, like almond milk. After you are on the detox for a bit, you can decide if you want to add the regular milk back in. If you do, make sure that you use it sparingly or not at all.

Some Things to Consider When You Are on a Detox

When you are ready to get started on a detox, there are a few things to consider. First, it is not just about the foods that you eat. You will also need to make some major lifestyle changes as well. Eating the right foods is the first step—but also consider having healthy relationships, drinking enough water, getting exercise, and getting enough sleep. If any of these points are missing, it can be really hard for the body to reduce the toxins.

First, make sure that you get enough sleep. Sleep is so important to help us function properly. You will have a hard time making it through the day and seeing the benefits of a detox if you are always sleepy. In addition, when you feel tired, it is harder than ever to avoid those sugar and carb cravings, and you will just give in and have trouble giving up. Try to aim for eight to nine hours of sleep a night, or add in a nap during the day, to help you get the most out of your detox plan.

Next, drink lots of water. Your body needs to have proper hydration, or it will run into issues with eliminating the toxins that you consume. This can assist the body more than anything else, and it is so simple to do. Aim for eight to ten glasses of water each day, and see what a difference it makes.

During the detox, you should aim to get a few minutes of exercise each day. You don't have to go crazy with it, but 30 minutes of moderate activity can be nice for the whole body. During the first few days of a sugar detox, it is fine to miss out on the exercise as your body adjusts to not having that steady stream of sugar available. Spend some time outside and walk around the blocks a few times on those days. But once you get through the crash, you can up the exercise a bit and then really see what the detox can do.

Finally, work on developing some healthy relationships in the process as well. If you are in a toxic relationship, or if you are constantly in and out of relationships, you may be used to falling back on comfort foods to help you feel better. If this sounds like something that you do, then it is time to fix your relationships before the detox. Good friends, ones who are there for you and support you, can push you so much further and can make the detox better. When you start out a new detox, consider whether you need a detox of the people around you as well.

Chapter 3: Simple Steps to Reduce Inflammation in the Body

Inflammation is a condition that many people suffer within their lives. It can make then uncomfortable, can make losing weight almost impossible, and can really add on pain if it is not managed. Many health conditions, including issues like arthritis, are caused by inflammation—and without taking the proper steps to deal with the inflammation, it can easily take over and cause your health to quickly deteriorate.

There are some steps that you can take to help reduce the amount of inflammation that is in the body. Choosing to eat a diet that is healthy and wholesome, one that gets rid of a lot of the bad stuff that you may currently eat can make a big difference. Let's look at some of the steps you can take to help reduce inflammation throughout the whole body.

Get Some Omega-3 Fatty Acids in Your Diet

The omega-3 fatty acids are so good for the body on so many different levels. First, EPA—one of the fatty acids of this kind found in fish oil, algae-based supplements, and fish, along with DHA—has properties to stop inflammation. You can get some of these from fish, but the right nutrients don't occur until the body converts them after eating. Also, these amounts are usually so small, that it isn't worth the effort.

Meanwhile, fish and fish oils can be a great way to get plenty of these omega-3 fatty acids into your diet plan. Try to get fresh fish into at least a few meals each day. If you aren't able to enjoy fish on a regular basis, consider starting a fish oil supplement so that you can get enough of these fatty acids to reduce inflammation throughout the body.

Eat Some Herbs

Herbs are not just great for adding some flavor to the foods you eat. If you eat the right ones, these herbs can help you reduce the amount of inflammation in the body. Some of the best herbs to consume include:

- Turmeric: This is a root that is bright orange, and it contains curcumin. Curcumin is going to help protect your liver from any cellular damage, and it can work as an antioxidant in the body to protect cells from free radical damage that causes inflammation. Add on that it helps lower histamine levels in the body, and you will quickly notice how the inflammation goes down.

- Ginger: Ginger has four important ingredients that can help reduce pain and reduce inflammation throughout the body. These ingredients—zingerone, shogaols, paradols, and gingerols—all work together to help you see a reduction in pain-inducing prostaglandins in the body.

- Cayenne: The heat that comes from cayenne can actually help reduce inflammation in the body. The capsaicin that is found in hot peppers and cayenne can help block the COX-2 enzyme, which will contribute to the inflammation process that can cause arthritis and other inflammatory diseases!

- Basil: Basil is a great herb to take in to help fight off inflammation. Eugenol is a compound found in basil, which gives it the smell that you recognize. It also helps reduce inflammation.

- White willow bark: This is a special type of bark that contains Salicin, which is related to some of the common ingredients found in Aspirin. The anti-inflammatory and pain relieving effects can actually last a lot longer than those in Aspirin, making it more effective.

- Oregano: Oregano has bioflavonoids and polyphenols, both of which are able to help fight off the free radicals in your body. This helps fight of inflammation throughout the whole body.

- Garlic: Garlic actually has a few different Sulphur compounds, which can make it a great option when reducing inflammation throughout the body. In addition, these compounds are going to fight off cancer and even reduce your risk of heart attack.

Be Careful About the Types of Fats You Consume

The types of fats that you consume in your diet can make a big influence on how much inflammation is in the body. First, let's take a look at those omega-6 fatty acids. These fatty acids are known for promoting inflammation throughout the body. They do this because these fats can help with the production of inflammatory compounds. And when the traditional American diet contains too many of these fats—found in options like cottonseed oils, soybean, and corn oils—you can imagine why inflammation is such a problem for many individuals.

Another fact that you need to watch out for when it comes to inflammation is trans-fat. These fats promote inflammation as well and can be found in products that use the words "partially hydrogenated oil" in its ingredient list. You will find a lot of these types of fats in foods like margarine, shortening, and baked goods so avoid these as much as possible is important.

This doesn't mean that you need to avoid all the fats in the world. In fact, some fats are important when it comes to helping the body absorb important nutrients from the other foods that you consume. However, you need to know which fats are bad for you and which ones promote your health—and Omega-6 fatty acids and trans-fats are *not* the good ones.

Refined Carbs and Sugars Are the Enemies

Sugars and refined carbs can contribute to a higher level of insulin and elevated blood sugars. This not only puts you at risk for diabetes—especially if the condition lasts for a long time—but it can also cause issues with inflammation in the body.

There are a number of bad things about all those sugars that you consume. They can contribute to a lot of weight gain and can make it difficult for someone to lose weight when they need. Not only are these carbs and sugars causing inflammation in the body, but extra body fat in the body is also contributing to the inflammation as well.

When you do pick out grains to eat (and these are allowed on most detoxes outside of juicing ones), make sure that they are whole grains. These are full of the healthy nutrients that your body needs, along with some really good carbs to keep the body running. They aren't going to get you on a bad carb cycle that is hard to get off. There are many great whole carb options that you can go with, including rice, bread, and pasta.

Eat Foods That Are Rich in Antioxidants

The biggest cause of inflammation throughout the body is free radicals floating around. These free radicals are considered compounds that are highly reactive. When you get too many inside the body, they can contribute to chronic inflammation while also causing damage to a lot of the cells in your body. Free radicals can get in your body from the environment, from what you eat, and from what you drink.

You can help clear the body of these free radicals, but you have to make sure you get the right nutrients in your diet. Antioxidants are able to neutralize these free radicals, which, in turn, helps reduce inflammation. Some of the antioxidants that you can use to help with this include vitamins A, C, and E. Where do you get these great antioxidants? They're from the fruits and vegetables, which should be on your plate during most detoxes.

To make sure that you are getting enough antioxidants in your diet, take a look at your plate. You want to see a lot of color there. If you see that a color is missing, you should make efforts to add it in. This variety in color helps you see your nutrients and ensures that you are covering all of your basis for nutrients throughout the day.

Take Some More Vitamin D in Your Diet

There are a lot of things that vitamin D is able to help you with. In this case, we are looking at how a deficiency in vitamin D can be associated with autoimmune conditions and inflammation. Some of the conditions that are affected by a deficiency in vitamin D include multiple sclerosis and Crohn's disease. The reason why vitamin D is so important has yet to be discovered, but the fact remains that your body really needs this nutrient.

There are two ways that you can take in enough vitamin D—either through the sun or through the food you eat. If you live in a warm climate, it is probably pretty easy to get outside and let the sun do its job providing you with vitamin D. However, for those who live in colder climates, vitamin D absorption from the sun is pretty hard to do.

If you aren't able to get enough vitamin D from the sun, then make sure you eat enough foods that are high in this nutrient. Options include almond and coconut milk, which have been fortified with vitamin D, fish, egg yolks, and other products that have added vitamin D into them.

What Do These All Have in Common?

We have discussed several different steps that you can take to help you reduce inflammation throughout the body. These steps are all effective, especially if you combine them together. But what do all of these have in common? They all rely on the diet you eat.

Most healthy detoxes are going to focus on the diets you consume. They understand that sometimes, changing the foods that you consume is enough to help you clean out the body and can help reduce the inflammation that you have throughout. Eating a diet that is low on sugars, high on fruits and vegetables, and even high on fish and other healthy products can really help reduce the inflammation in your whole body.

When you eat a diet that is high on poor nutrients, your body is going to react with a lot of inflammation. This is why you may have issues with irritable bowel syndrome, arthritis, and more. The bad fats and sugars in your body and the lack of good nutrition is what is causing this inflammation. The longer you stick with that poor diet, the worse the problem with inflammation is going to get for you.

However, you can make a change. Getting rid of those bad foods, especially the sugars and the refined carbs—and focusing more on eating foods that are healthy and wholesome, like lots of fresh fruits and vegetables—can be the thing you need to solve this problem. Try going even five days with no sugar or refined carbs and plenty of fruits and vegetables and whole grains, and see if the pain from inflammation, along with other serious health conditions, will go away for you!

Many people are looking for ways to reduce the amount of inflammation that is in their bodies. They may be tired of the pain and the other health conditions that this inflammation can cause if it is not treated. Simply changing around the diet you consume can be enough to make inflammation a thing of the past. Rather than relying on medications and other treatments that are hard and expensive, consider changing up the diet you eat and let your body naturally heal all on its own.

Chapter 4: Improving Your Immune System Through a Detox

Your immune system is very important. It is there to help you keep the body strong, to help you avoid any of those bugs that go around during the winter time. When the immune system isn't doing its best work, you are going to feel it. You may feel down and tired and like you have a constant cold, and you may have to deal with issues of staying in bed and missing work.

Changing up the diet that you eat can make a big difference in your overall health. When you cut out the sugars and the processed foods and instead choose to focus on foods that are good and wholesome for you, it becomes much easier to keep the body healthy. All that fresh fruits and vegetables, all that healthy whole grains, and all those lean sources of protein can flood your body with the nutrients it needs to stay healthy.

What is truly amazing is that a healthy immune system can actually help improve so many different aspects of your life. Are you dealing with inflammation? It could be from your immune system reacting to the free radicals in the body. Dealing with stomach issues, the immunity could be causing some chaos there as well.

This is why it is so important that when you go on a detox—you make sure you also work on eating foods that are good for your whole immune system as well. The good news is that if you go on a sugar detox and work to reduce how much sugar you consume each day, you are going to automatically start eating foods that are better for your system.

Foods That Clean Out the Body

When you are worried about your immune system and how it functions, you need to make sure that you are cleaning out the body as much as possible. There are a lot of foods that tend to gunk up the immune system and make it work a lot harder than it needs to. When the body is busy dealing with chronic illnesses and busy fighting off those free radicals, it has a hard time focusing on getting rid of any cold or flu, or any other disease, that happens to come around.

The first thing that you need to do, hopefully long before you get sick, is learning how to clean out the body and prevent it from getting all messed up again. There are many foods you can rely on that will help you get that immune system in order and will ensure that your body stays as healthy as possible. Some of the best foods to enjoy that will also help clean out the body include:

- Apples: The pectin that is found in apples is perfect for cleaning out the intestines and making your stomach happier.
- Avocados: These are a popular food source, but most people do not consider them as a cleansing food. They do a lot of good in the body when it comes to dilating the blood vessels and lowering cholesterol. They also have a nutrient inside them known as glutathione, which is able to block out a ton of carcinogens while helping the liver detoxify.

- Beets: Beets contain a unique mixture of natural plant compounds that help make them perfect for cleaning out the blood and the liver.

- Blueberries: These are one of the best healing foods because they have a ton of antioxidants and they have a natural aspirin inside that can reduce inflammation and lessen pain in the body. They also contain a type of antibiotic that will help prevent infections in the urinary tract.

- Cabbage: Cabbage has a lot of antioxidant and anticancer compounds, and it is a good one for helping the liver break down some of the extra hormones that are there. Cabbages can also help clean out the digestive tract so your stomach can absorb other nutrients better.

- Celery and celery seeds: These are great cleaners for the blood, and they will help detoxify the cancer cells that are in the body. They also help because they contain more than twenty substances that can reduce inflammation.

- Cranberries: If you are dealing with an infection of any kind, it may be time to look at cranberries. These cranberries include antibiotic and antiviral substances that can clean out the body.

- Kale: Steam up some kale to help benefit the whole body. This food can help clean out the whole body from a variety of harmful substances. It also has a high level of fiber that can clean out the intestinal tract.

- Lemons: Lemons are a great way to detoxify the liver, and they have a lot of vitamin C to help fight off illness.

- Seaweed: This may not be a type of food that you are used to dealing with, but it could really help when you are fighting off illness. According to studies that were done at the McGill University of Montreal, seaweed can bind to the radioactive waste inside the body. It can also bind to heavy metals that are in the body and will eliminate them.

These are just a few of the different food types that you can include in your diet in order to see your body cleaned out and to help you suffer from less inflammation and fewer illnesses because of the immune system. The most important thing that you can do here is to pick out a lot of variety in your meals, focusing mainly on some good herbs and fresh produce. If you can fill up your plate with a lot of healthy and wholesome foods, then it is easy to keep the immune system running strong.

The Best Foods for Boosting Your Immune System

There are a ton of different foods that you can eat that will help you get the right nutrition to keep that immune system up and running. In the next section, we are going to explore some of the different nutrients that are important to your immune system, but some of the foods you can enjoy to get these nutrients include the following:

- Citrus fruits: These contain a ton of vitamin C, which can help increase the production of white blood cells throughout the body.

- Red bell peppers: Once for ounce, red bell peppers are going to contain twice as much vitamin C as citrus. They also contain a lot of beta-carotene that helps as well. Also, they will help you get healthy skin and eyes in the process.

- Broccoli: Broccoli contains the right amounts of vitamins A, C, and E and other antioxidants to keep the body working strong. The key here is to make sure you cook the broccoli as little as possible, or some of the nutrients will seep out.

- Yogurt: Look for yogurts that have something about live and active cultures on them. Greek yogurt is a good example. Get ones that are plain, and then add in some fruits if you light to help avoid some of the unhealthy sugars that can harm the immune system.

- Almonds: When it comes to fighting off—or even preventing a cold—vitamin E is often forgotten, but it is very important. It is a fat-soluble vitamin that needs fat to help it absorb properly. Nuts, like almonds, have the fats that this vitamin needs to be absorbed and get all the health benefits as well.

- Green tea: Both the green and black teas are going to be packed up with flavonoids, an antioxidant that can clear out the body and help protect the immune system all at once.
- Kiwi: Kiwis are naturally full of a lot of essential nutrients, many of the ones we talk about below, that you should keep a few nearby when cold and flu season comes around.

Your Ultimate Nutrition and Vitamins Plan

A healthy immune system is so important to the overall functioning of our bodies. We want to be able to get through our lives without having to spend too many days on the couch because we are sick. However, when you don't give your body enough nutrients to thrive, the immune system may be the first to go. This doesn't mean that those who eat a lot of fruits and vegetables will never get sick—but it does mean that they will get sick a lot less often than others do.

Many people don't eat enough of the vegetables, fruits, and other foods that are needed in order to keep them healthy throughout the whole year. You can't sit there and eat one orange or one apple and expect the vitamin C from that to prevent that cold from hitting you. A truly healthy immune system is going to depend on a balanced mix of vitamins and minerals over time, along with some exercise and normal sleep patterns. When you can get all of these to work together, your immune system will be healthier than ever.

Whenever you can, it is best to get your vitamins and minerals from food, rather than relying on a pill to provide for you. If you live in an area where fresh fruits and where vegetables were hard to come by, or you are worried about some gaps in your nutrient when you first start, then you can consider a multivitamin to supplement. However, never rely on this as the full dosage of vitamins for you.

Now, there are several different types of vitamins and minerals that the immune system needs to thrive. Most of us just think about vitamin C, but there are actually quite a few others that you need as well. Let's take a look at some of the best vitamins and minerals that you can take to help keep your immune system strong.

Vitamin C

First on the list is vitamin C. When most people think about their immune system, they automatically think about vitamin C. There are a lot of places where you can get plenty of vitamin C, though, which should make it easier for you to get enough. Some options that you can choose are papaya, strawberries, Brussels sprouts, bell peppers, kale, and spinach. In fact, there are so many foods that contain this vitamin, that it is not really one that you need to supplement, especially if you are on a detox.

Vitamin E

Just like with vitamin C, vitamin E is considered an antioxidant that will help the body fight off infections. Sunflower seeds, hazelnuts, peanuts, and almonds are all high in this vitamin. You can even get this one through broccoli and spinach if you prefer to increase your intake through meals.

Vitamin A

Vitamin A is the next nutrient on the list when it comes to a healthy immune system. When you are looking for vitamin A, make sure that you find foods that have a lot of color, such as squash, pumpkin, sweet potatoes, and carrots. These all contain carotenoids, which the body is able to convert over to vitamin A. They also have a nice antioxidant effect that will strengthen the immune system against infection.

Vitamin D

We talked about this vitamin a bit before when we were exploring inflammation, but it is also important when it comes to the health of your immune system. It is best to get your vitamins from food, but this one is an exception to this rule. For this one, it is easiest and often best to get the nutrient from the sun. But for those who live in colder climates and who have to bundle up through most of the year, this is easier said than done.

There are a few different ways that you can increase your consumption of vitamin D. You can find it in fatty fish, such as sardines, tuna, mackerel, and salmon—as well as in foods that are fortified with it, such as milk, cereals, and orange juice. If you still have trouble getting in enough vitamin D to your diet, consider talking with your doctor about taking some supplements to help.

Folate or folic acid

Folate is the natural form of this nutrient while folic acid is known as the synthetic form. These two nutrients are often added to foods because there aren't a ton of foods that have them, and they are really beneficial to the body, especially when you are pregnant and for your developing baby.

To get more folate, you should try to add in lots of leafy green vegetables and peas and beans to your plate on a regular basis. You can also look for some fortified foods to see if they contain more of this folic acid. Read the labels to check, but lots of whole grain products, like cereal, pasta, rice, and enriched bread will add in some folic acid.

Iron

Next on the list is iron. Iron is in charge of carrying oxygen to all of the cells. You can find iron in many different forms. Your body can absorb what is known as the "heme iron" the easiest. You can find this form of iron in foods such as turkey, chicken, and seafood. If you are following a vegetarian diet, you can still find this form of iron if you look through kale, broccoli, and beans.

Selenium

Selenium has a really powerful effect on the immune system. To start, selenium has a powerful effect on the immune system, including its potential to slow down how the body reacts to certain aggressive cancers. You can find this nutrient in many locations include barley, brazil nuts, tuna, sardines, broccoli, and garlic.

Zinc

There are many places where you can find plenty of zinc. Take a look at chickpeas, yogurt, baked beans (just make sure you get the kind without added sugar, lean meat and poultry, crab, and oysters. Zinc is a good nutrient to get into your body because it can help slow down how quickly the immune system will respond to control any inflammation that is occurring in the body. This can help give you a bit of relief from the pain.

Fresh fruits and vegetables are often the best when it comes to getting nutrients to boost the immune system. However, if you need to get some produce that isn't available in the regular aisle, or you need it to last a little bit longer, then it is fine to work with frozen produce as well.

Your immune system is a very important part of your overall health. It helps keep inflammation away, can keep you from getting sick, and can reduce a lot of the other health conditions that are in your body. Make sure to follow the advice in this chapter so that you can see the results of how well foods and your diet can impact inflammation.

Chapter 5: Ending Your Sugar and Carb Cravings

As we have discussed in this guidebook, sugars can be the enemy. While they taste good and we all enjoy having something that is full of refined carbs and sugar, the negatives to our health far outweigh the temporary feelings of happiness and satisfaction that we may get from consuming lots of sugars. Going on a sugar detox and getting rid of all the sugars and the refined carbs in our diet can be one of the best ways to reset the metabolism and the taste buds so that you can finally break free of this addiction.

Now, you may understand why you need to get rid of some of the sugars, but why are we including refined carbs in here? Refined carbs are going to include options like white bread, white pasta, and pretty much anything that is made with white flour. The problem with these is that when the body digests and absorbs them, they will also be converted into glucose, just like sugar does, in the body. When you combine a diet high in sugar with a diet high in refined carbs, you are taking in way more glucose than the body needs. Also, all that extra glucose that isn't used by the cells as energy will be stored as body fat, usually around the belly.

This is why when we choose to go on a sugar detox, we are going to choose to cut out both sugars and refined carbs. Cutting these both down, especially by the large amounts that the sugar detox wants, will make a big difference. Keep in mind that we are talking about refined carbs here. Whole grains and whole wheat carbs are fine, as are the complex carbs that are found in fruits and vegetables. Those options are just fine when you are on a sugar detox.

Now that we understand a bit more about starting with a sugar detox and the different foods that can help with your immune system and inflammation, let's take a look at some of the basics that come with choosing a sugar detox.

Why Are We Addicted to Sugar?

Those cravings for sugar can actually show that we are addicted to sugar. Many scientists believe that we are primed to desire sugar on an almost instinctive level because it used to play an important role in our survival. Our sense of taste has evolved to covet the molecules vital to life like fat and salt. When we eat something, the glucose will be absorbed from the intestines into the bloodstream and then distributed to all the other cells of the body. This glucose is really important to the brain because it provides a lot of fuel to all the neuronal nerve cells there.

These neurons need a constant supply of glucose from the bloodstream because while they need this glucose to work, they aren't able to make it themselves. As a diabetic knows all too well, when someone with low blood sugar isn't able to get glucose quickly, they can go into a coma.

Even the taste of sugar can really boost the brain. Some studies and tests have been done and show that participants who swill water that is sweetened by sugar in their mouths were able to perform better on a mental task than when they gargle artificially sweetened water.

The relationship that we have with sugar is going to start at birth. A study published from Washington University found that newborns have a preference for sweet flavors over all others, while children are going to enjoy foods with sugar more than adults. Many believe that this preference for sweet things is an evolutionary gene. In the past, younger children who preferred foods with high calories would have survived better when food became scarce or unreliable.

Eating all this sugar can lead to unhealthy eating patterns. This sugar can boost the mood, and it will prompt the body to release the happy hormone—also known as serotonin—into the blood. The boost that we get from sugar is one of the reasons that people turn to this when they are celebrating or when they need a reward or a comfort. However, when you have this pleasant rush, it is going to increase your insulin, as the body strives to get your glucose levels back to normal. This can cause you to have a sugar crash, resulting in more cravings for more sugar, and the process goes on and on.

In addition, our bodies are not able to tell when we have taken in enough, or too much, sugar. Researchers found that drinks and food sweetened with fructose do not trigger the same sense of fullness as other foods that have similar calories. One study that was done by Yale University found that while glucose was able to suppress the parts of the brain that make us hungry, fructose didn't. In the test, the participants often reported feeling more satisfied when they consumed glucose compared to those taking in fructose. Since many processed foods are sweetened by sucrose, which contains 50 percent fructose, eating a lot of these types of foods can make it hard to resist the cravings.

However, the body is not able to tell the difference between natural sugars, like those found in milk, honey, and fruit, and processed sugars from baked goods, candy and more. All sugars will be broken down in the body into fructose and glucose and then they are processed by the liver. The sugars can then be converted over into glycogen or fat for storage—or the glucose in the blood for use in the body's cells.

The body does use up the glucose, as long as you don't take in too many. And when you eat the unhealthy types of sugars, like fructose, it is hard to stop. You still feel hungry, you have lots of cravings, and you can't turn it off. But when all that glucose is in the body, you won't be able to use it all up and it gets stored as belly fat, which can make it possible for many chronic health illnesses to affect you.

There are a lot of reasons that sugar can be bad for the body. Also, the more sugars that you take in, the worse the problem can be. Some of the most common health concerns for those who take in too much sugar include:

- Causes weight gain
- Increases your risk of heart disease
- Can increase how much acne you have.
- Increases the risk of diabetes.
- Can increase how likely you are to get cancer
- Can cause issues with depression
- May accelerate the aging process of your skin
- Can increase cellular aging
- Drains your energy
- Can lead to fatty liver disease

These are just some of the common health concerns that you may face when you eat too much sugar. And when you get into the vicious cycle with not being able to stop your sugar addiction, things are just going to get worse. This is where a sugar detox can come into play.

A sugar detox can help this. By eliminating the sugars completely and working through the cravings, you can then reset your eating habits. This can break that vicious cycle and will ensure that you can give up those sugars and reduce some of the bad health results that are listed above.

There are different forms of a sugar detox. Some people just give up processed sugars and sugars that are found in fast foods, processed foods, and baked goods, for example. Others will focus on getting rid of all sugars, such as fruits and dairy products because they want to really kick-start their detox and ensure that they can get rid of the cravings.

Either way, you can finally break the habit of being addicted to sugar. You just need to eat a diet that is full of healthy and wholesome foods. You can choose to add another diet plan to this, or you can just eat foods that are going to provide your body with all the nutrients it needs.

How to Go on a Sugar Detox

Let's break down the process you need to go on in order to end your sugar cravings and help you finally get on a healthier lifestyle. We are going to break it down by days a bit so that you can see what steps are needed and to ensure you can actually see results.

The day before you start a detox, take some time to go through the house and your kitchen. Get rid of anything that has processed sugars and refined carbs in them, and then throw them out. Afterward, hit the grocery store and stock up on lots of wholesome foods and options. If you need to, consider setting up a meal plan during the few days before the detox. Freezer meals or slow cooker meals can be nice with this. Then, when you are having a craving or dealing with a busy or stressful night, you can just grab out a healthy supper and be ready to go with no preparation that evening.

Day 1: Cut out all sugars that you have in your diet.

This is considered a pure sugar detox, which means that you need to completely cut out everything that has sugar. This detox has to remove all of the artificial sugars from your diet. One way to ensure that you are eliminating the right sugars is to look at the ingredients, or the label, and avoid anything that states it is low sugar. This usually means that the manufacturer cut down on sugars, but they added in more fats or sodium in order to help with the flavor. They may also add in sugar alcohols, which aren't much better.

During this time, it is fine to eat whole foods that have some natural sugars, which means fruits. If this is still a trigger for you (which it is for some people with sugar addiction), then cut out fruits for the first few days as well. You should fill your plate up with whole grains, lean cuts of meat, and lots of vegetables (and fruits if you want to include them) to provide your body with the nutrition that it needs.

Day 3 to 7: Concentrate on eating healthy snacks to help with withdrawal symptoms.

When you are stopping sugar in this detox, the first three days or so are going to be the hardest for everyone. You may have several symptoms of withdrawal including sugar cravings, muscle aches, headaches, and fatigue. Some people have trouble sleeping, shaking, nausea, lack of focus, and dizziness.

Then, after the five days are done, you may start to feel lighter. This is an important stage where you need to eat whole grains, healthy snacks, and lots of greens to help minimize the cravings for sugars. Your body may spend this time crying out for food, and you need to fill it with these good things to fill it up and keep your blood sugars balanced. As soon as those blood sugar levels become unbalanced, your cravings will get much worse, so having healthy snacks on hand will make a difference.

Day 8 to 10: At this point, the sugar is out of your system. You should be able to taste the difference.

Once you have gotten through the week, you are going to feel a bit more focused, and you will notice that your cognitive functioning is improving compared to earlier in the detox. Depending on the person, this sometimes happens after just four days on the detox.

Then, after ten days have passed, the taste buds are going to start to change, and you are basically resetting the whole system. Sugar, as well as its taste, will signal the hormonal system so that it knows when it is time for the body needs to eat. If you were successful with the sugar detox, the cravings are going to end, and you may have a lower tolerance for sweetness compared to before. There may even be times when you think a food is too sweet. Make sure that you don't give in to temptation now. Just keep eating meals that are healthy and home cooked so that you don't reset yourself.

Day 15 to 21: This is the time when you can start adding in some sugars to the diet, one by one.

After you reach the 15-day mark, your energy is going to be back at its peak. You will be more aware of the digestion process and now that you have been able to eliminate the effects of sugar on the system, you will be better equipped to identify satisfying foods and those that cause some inflammation.

During this week, you are going to start feeling better. You will have more energy and you can better identify hunger pains and sugar cravings. This is a crucial period for those who are always busy because they may have had trouble doing this in the past when they were always running.

You can slowly start to add more of the sugars into your diet. If you got rid of all sugars, such as those from milk and fruits, this is when you can start to add them back in, along with a few desserts here and there. Take it slowly though. Introduce one food back into the diet every few days. You may find that you have a slight intolerance to something, such as milk, and will want to completely get rid of using it. Or, you may find that the desserts you used to love are now too sweet.

After the sugar detox, you can slowly start eating things that weren't allowed on the meal plan. Make sure that you don't over indulge with this or you may feel very uncomfortable or can start to put yourself back into the vicious cycle with sugar. It is fine to have some sugar, just make sure that you are portioning out the food the right way. And once you are done eating something that is sweet, make sure that you consume something that contains whole grains, lean protein, and fiber.

Tips to Make a Sugar Detox Easier

Giving up sugar is hard. We like to have sugar. It tastes good and can even make us temporarily feel better after we eat it, and our bodies crave it more than anything else. Giving up this sugar is not always easy when the good tastes and our bodies are fighting against us. Here are a few tips that you can follow in order to make a sugar detox easier.

- Cut it all out at once: Some people recommend that you cut out one thing at a time and slowly get rid of sugar. This can work for some, but for others, they will simply substitute one missing sugar with another. It is often best to just cut out everything and get through the hard part all at once. This gives your body time to recover from the sugar and can make it easier to get through the cravings part. It will be tough for a few days, but much better than drawing the process out.

- Get plenty of protein in your day: Protein should be found during every meal, especially at breakfast after fasting all night. This helps balance out your blood sugars and can cut out cravings. Consider a protein shake or a whole egg meal to make this work.

- Fight off the sugar craving with some fat: Fat is not always the enemy hear. Fat is going to make you full, can balance out your blood sugars, and can be necessary for fueling up the cells. Along with plenty of protein, good fats should be present as much as possible in all your snacks and meals.

- Be ready when an emergency happens: You never want to end up in a food emergency when the blood sugar is dropping. Then, you may make your way to a vending machine, a fast food restaurant, or a convenience store. These are going to have a bunch of the refined carbs and sugars that you need to avoid during this time. Keeping a few snacks in your purse or in the car can help tide you over until you can get home. Fill them with snacks that have good fats and protein so that you won't be tempted to make a bad choice.

- Swap out distress for de-stress: If you feel stressed out, the hormones are going to go crazy. Cortisol will go up, causing you to feel hungry (even if you aren't), causing belly fat storage that can eventually lead to type-2 diabetes. Studies show that finding methods to relax, such as deep breathing, can help move you out of the stress state and can help you avoid the hormones all going crazy. A simple method is a five-breath break. Before each meal, simply take five slow and deep breaths, going to a count of five in and five out. This will make a big difference in how much you actually eat when you sit down.

- Get rid of the inflammation: Studies have shown how inflammation can trigger some imbalances in blood sugar, pre-diabetes, insulin resistance, and type-2 diabetes. The most common source of inflammatory foods, outside of sugar, are trans-fat and flour. When you cut out some of these bad things, you can get rid of the inflammation and have a healthier lifestyle.

- Get enough sleep: I can't emphasize this one enough. When you don't provide the body with enough sleep, it can drive your carbs and sugar cravings because it affects the appetite hormones. In human studies, when college students were deprived of just two hours of sleep, their hunger hormones increased, and they saw a decrease in the appetite-suppressing hormones. These college students also started to have more cravings for refined carbs and sugar. Sleep is the best way to help you prevent overeating and can help make your weight and your cravings go away.

A sugar detox is one of the best things that you can do for your overall health. It will help you get rid of the cravings for sugar, help you eat healthier and can put a bunch of chronic health problems at bay. Following the advice in this chapter will make it easier for you to really get a good start on your own sugar detox.

Chapter 6: Easy Habits That You Can Adopt to Kick Those Sugar Cravings Out

Fighting off that sugar craving can seem almost impossible. Our bodies want to hold onto the sugar because it can be a potential energy source later. But since we aren't running away from animals or going through long periods of famine in our modern times, that sugar carving can lead to a lot of health problems and can make us really sick. The good news is that there are a few easy habits that you can implement into your schedule to help you finally kick those sugar cravings to the curb including:

Replace Your Evening Snack with a Fruit

Late night snacking is a hard thing to beat. You may have done well all day long, but once you finally get some time to relax and put your feet up, you are ready for a nice sugary snack. It is hard to give up this. Some people may try. But for those who just can't give up that habit, it is important to have some other options available.

One thing to consider is to substitute that sugary snack with some fruit. An apple or a banana can provide your body with a little bit of natural sugar so that you can help that craving, without giving in completely. That apple at night is much better than that candy bar or that big piece of cake. It contains the natural sugar, which is better than what is found in desserts, along with healthy vitamins and nutrients. This all comes together to help keep the body strong and to keep you away from those cravings.

Plan Out Your Meals Ahead of Time

Planning out your meals ahead of time and making sure that you don't get too hungry can make a big difference in how many cravings you have. First, let's look at planning out your meals. You should plan at least a week in advance, though some people like to go further than that. You can get all the ingredients for your meals and snacks and know that they are healthy. If you take this far enough, you can even do freezer meals, which help you get a healthy dinner on the table in just a few minutes, even on those nights when you are really busy.

The more you leave things to chance, the harder it is to avoid those cravings. If you get home from a long day of work and then sports events with the kids, how likely are you to make a delicious and healthy home cooked meal when you have to start from scratch? It is likely that you will reach for something out of the freezer, something full of sugars and refined carbs, which will make the craving worse later.

Always plan out your meals, and try not to go too long between meals before you eat again. This helps you avoid those cravings because you are famished at the end of the day. You can utilize your Instant Pot, your slow cooker, or make a bunch of freezer meals. Just make sure that you have a plan to help you avoid those cravings.

Clean Out the Kitchen to Avoid Temptations

If there is something sugary around your home, you are more likely to reach for it and eat it up as soon as you get a craving. It is really hard to avoid a temptation when it is right in your home. One of the best ways to avoid this temptation is to go through and clean your kitchen, getting rid of all the sugary foods that can cause those cravings and replacing them with healthier options.

Set aside a few hours and look through everything in your kitchen. Look at labels and decide what has a lot of refined carbs and sugars inside it and toss out anything that will make your cravings worse. You may be surprised at how many things you will kick out of your cupboards during this time.

When you are done, it is time to head to the grocery store. You still have to eat something, and with the cupboards bare, it is time to go through and replace all those bad foods with something good. If you are going on a detox, make sure to pick up foods that fit with that option. Otherwise, replace those bad foods with lean meats, lots of fresh produce, legumes, and whole grains to keep you full and the sugar cravings at bay.

Drink Some Water When You Have a Craving

One of the biggest reasons that you are craving something salty or sugary is because you are thirsty. The first thing that you should do when you feel that a craving is coming up is to drink a glass of water. It could be that the body is trying to tell you it is thirsty, but we assume that it is hungry and we eat something that is not good for us. Make sure to keep plenty of water nearby for those times when you feel a craving but aren't that hungry, and see what a difference it can make.

Eat Healthy Meals

No matter how you look at it, chocolate chips and other candy can be really tasty. And when you are really hungry, your body may instantly try to crave something that is that tasty. The trick to fight against this is to eat healthy meals on a regular basis. Yes, when we are busy with our modern lives, it is sometimes easier to skip meals, but it is still important to eat meals that are healthy so that you don't become too ravenous.

The hungrier you get, the more powerless you become against those sugar cravings later. Even if you have to bring a small snack around you on those busy days when you just can't get to a meal, make sure that you don't go too long without eating to avoid those cravings.

The healthy meals that you eat need to contain some lean meats, lots of fresh produce (especially those vegetables), some whole grains (stay away from all the white and refined grains), and some healthy dairy if you choose to add it in. When you combine these together, you will be able to provide your body with all the nutrients it needs, along with plenty of satiety that can help keep the sugar cravings away.

Identify Your Triggers

Many people have triggers that make them start craving sugars more than usual. Aside from some of the physical reasons for craving sugar, such as being overly hungry and being dehydrated, the reason that you are craving these foods can be virtually anything and each person is different. If you are someone who is prone to these cravings, it is important to take a look at your feelings and thoughts when the cravings strike.

Over time, you will be able to identify a pattern. Sometimes the key to getting through the craving is not to fight it but to deal with the underlying cause itself. You may crave sugars when you are stressed out, when you are feeling down, or when you are tired. You can learn how to avoid these triggers and see some great results with your health as well. If you are tired, you maybe need to consider going to bed earlier or take a nap during the day. If you eat when you are stressed, consider new ways, such as exercising and meditation, to help reduce your stress. Each trigger has a way to solve it—you just need to learn what yours I and then work from there.

Take In Enough Complex Carbs

Just like dehydration can cause some food cravings, having a lack of healthy carbs can cause you to crave sugar as well. Realize that there is a difference in the types of carbs that you can eat. Don't go reaching for the processed or refined carbs. These are basically sugar in disguise and will do nothing to help you avoid that sugar craving. But if you focus on eating whole grains and other complex carbs, like those found in fruits and vegetables, you can easily kick that sugar craving away.

There are a lot of great complex carbs that you can choose from. Some of the best options that will make that sugar craving go away and can fill you up include peas, lentils, beans, pasta, whole grain bread, green vegetables, and sweet potatoes. These are able to provide the body with some energy that will last a lot longer than what the simple or refined carbs can give, along with a lot of nutrients and vitamins.

Yes, there are times when you may have a craving for a simple carb, like a sweet treat, but it is amazing how quickly the body can burn through those and how hungry you are going to feel in a short amount of time—and those sugars will make you crave more of the sugars and raise your insulin levels and blood sugar levels.

Conclusion

Thank you for making it through to the end of *Sugar Detox*. Let's hope it was informative and able to provide you with all of the tools you need to achieve your goals, whatever they may be.

Sugar is all around us. It is hard to avoid. Many times, we are eating more sugar than we realize because it was added in without us knowing. Reading labels, knowing what foods contain how much sugar, and really being a smart consumer about our health and the foods that we eat is the best way to ensure we get foods that are good and healthy for us.

This guidebook has the goal of helping you understand why sugar is so bad, why you need to avoid it, and why it is sometimes so hard to avoid sugar in the first place. In the past, our ancestors had to rely on sugar to keep them from starving. Sugars were a good source of energy, one that could be stored until later and then used up during a famine or longer periods of time without food. Eating a bunch when available was a way to survive.

But today, this is not true. Many of us live in a world of abundance—one where we can get food, including sugar, any time that we want. But that primal urge to eat as much sugar as we can, just in case of a famine, is still there, and it can be really hard to beat and to ignore.

This guidebook gave you the tools that you need to stop relying so much on sugars and refined carbs. We talked about the importance of a detox to clean out the body and why sugars can be so bad for the body—and then provided you with a sugar detox that will make all the difference in your health. Sure, it may be hard to go on one of these detoxes in the beginning, but the hard part will soon pass, and you will feel the energy, the better outlook on life, and all the health benefits.

Reducing and eliminating sugars and refined carbs out of your diet can effectively help every aspect of your health. It starts with helping your immune system and reducing inflammation throughout the body. Both of these come together and form the basis of many serious health conditions when they aren't working properly. Too many sugars can throw them off and cause illnesses, while a detox can clear up that issue and help you get your health back on track.

A detox doesn't have to be scary, and it doesn't have to mess with your whole lifestyle. It is meant to be a way to clear up the body and get you in the best shape of your life—with less pain, less inflammation, and fewer illnesses than before. This guidebook will provide you with all the information that you need to get started with a sugar detox today!

Finally, if you found this book useful in any way, a review on Amazon is always appreciated!

Fatty Liver Diet:

Guide on How to End Fatty Liver Disease

Introduction

Taking an active role in your health is important. If you are worried about your liver, you may have heard about doing a liver detox, cleanse or flush. Your liver, the second largest organ in your body, processes external medicine and internal nutrients in addition to making sure your body removes potentially harmful toxins. Many people decide to do a liver detox after extended consumption of processed foods alcohol in order to assist their body in removing these toxins. Other people turn to a liver detox to assist their daily life. Additionally, others consider a liver detox when they have developed a liver disease and are looking for additional treatment options.

Similar to other detoxes, there are variations available and certain things you need to know before beginning. For example, there are **different foods and drinks that are good for supporting your liver's** health, and other foods and drinks that can be harmful. Some detoxes are best for a single day while others can last up to a week or more. Some are actually very unhealthy for your body while others support your nutritional needs. These are just some of the reasons why you need to pay attention to what you choose to do to detox your liver and also support your overall health.

Detoxing your liver helps you in a variety of ways. First, you will most likely begin to feel better early in the process. You will feel lighter, healthier, and energetic. Second, you will help your body begin to adjust to a healthy diet instead of existing on unhealthy foods and drinks. Finally, you will begin to remove excess toxins and fat build up from your body.

The reason you experience these amazing benefits is that a liver detox, especially ones focused on your over health and liver function, removes processed foods and alcohol from your diet for a period of time. Foods and drinks in these categories are high-calorie, high-sugar, and high-fat foods that do not deliver a proportional level of nutrients. Other benefits include a focus on whole foods which means many foods people are sensitive to are removed. For example, most detoxes require you to cease eating gluten-rich foods and dairy.

Your liver is critically important to the function of your body, and doing a liver detox is a great natural way to support healthy liver function and heal damage to your liver. It is not always possible to repair existing damage, but detoxes can prevent future damage and support your general health in the meantime.

Doctors say liver detoxes aren't important for your health or how well your liver works. There's no proof they help get rid of toxins after you've had too much food or alcohol. There's also no evidence that they fix the liver damage that has already happened.

A Few Things to Know About the Safety of Liver Detoxes

If you already have a liver disease, you are should be working closely with your medical team to treat your liver. Talk with them about a liver cleanse and make sure to remain under their supervision while completing the detox. Make sure you choose a detox that is good for you with a focus on nutrition and health instead of weight loss or chemical additives. Other considerations include:

- Beware of liver-detox products available for sale in a store. These can contain harmful ingredients and also may make false claims regarding the safety and effectiveness of the product.
- A juice that is unpasteurized has the potential to make you ill. The risk increases for people who have a weak immune system and also for the elderly.
- Other illnesses can be made worse by a liver detox. For example, a 24-hour liver detox juice cleanse can irritate and worsen a pre-existing kidney disease. Fasting before or during the detox can worsen hepatitis B. If you have any other illnesses and are considering doing a liver detox, make sure to talk with your medical professional about any potential conflicts with doing the detox.
- Diabetes is another disease that requires medical intervention and supervision. Again, make sure you work with your medical team to make sure your detox does not interfere with any other medical condition, like diabetes.
- Side effects including dehydration, headaches, light-headed, or weakness, can occur, especially if you choose to fast as part of the process.

Keep Your Liver Healthy

Your liver's health is determined by your genetics and general health. Your environment, lifestyle, and diet also affect your liver's health. There are things you can do before, during and after your detox to help support your overall health and your liver health. Some of the following guidelines are beneficial, especially if you are predisposed to the liver disease. For example, a history of liver disease in your family or excessive alcohol consumption can make it more likely that you develop the fatty liver disease. The guidelines are as follows:

1. Cut back on your alcohol consumption.
2. Every day, focus on eating a diet that is well balanced. This includes protein, whole grains, seeds, nuts, fresh vegetables, and fruits.
3. Obtain and maintain a healthy weight for your age, gender, and height.
4. Try to get moderate to high levels of exercise every day. If you have been inactive or only minimally active, make sure to work with your medical professional before adopting any new lifestyle change.
5. Hepatitis is very dangerous to your general health but especially harmful to your liver. Minimize the likelihood of contracting hepatitis by:

    a. Avoid unprotected sex with people you do not know well.
    b. Patronize reputable and sterile tattoo parlors for any tattoo you get.
    c. Use your own personal household items, toothbrushes, and razors.
    d. Do not use illegal drugs. If you decide to utilize them, do not share straws or needles with others.

The Main Reasons for Completing a Liver Detox for Preventing and Curing Fatty Liver Disease

1. **Lose weight.**

Bile is what removes fat and toxins from your body and your liver produces bile. This means, in order to lose weight, you need to produce enough bile to get it out of your body. If you have been struggling with losing weight, this could be the reason.

2. **Remove liver stones.**

Your lover does not just build up fat; it can also build up cholesterol. This creates liver stones and that can be incredibly painful and detrimental to your health.

3. **Overall body detox and health support.**

When you do a detox, you remove toxins from your body. Any excess toxins can harm your body in multiple places. This is why a liver detox promotes your health in all areas.

4. **Improves energy levels.**

5. **The liver moves toxins out and nutrients through your body.**

When it does not function properly due to fat buildup, nutrients may not be making it into your bloodstream as you need. This can make you feel sluggish and fatigued. When you get your liver functioning again, it is likely the increase in nutrients reaching your body will also boost your energy levels.

6. **Makes your appear and feel younger.**

Your liver affects the health and appearance of your skin. When your liver is healthy, your skin looks and feels healthier. This external improvement helps you look and feel younger.

Chapter 1: What Is Fatty Liver Disease?

Simply defined, the fatty liver disease is a liver condition caused by a fat buildup in the organ. The human body has only one other organ that is larger than the liver, skin, and no internal organs larger than the liver. The many functions of the liver include disposing of harmful toxins, processing fat from the bloodstream and helping in the blood clotting function.

When the liver stops working correctly, fat begins to build up. Some of the reasons the liver stops working correctly include alcohol, hepatitis C, reactions to various medications, and rare metabolic issues. Conditions during pregnancy can also cause fat build up in the liver for women. There is a special category designated for other situations that lead to fat build up in the liver; NAFLD or Non-Alcoholic Fatty Liver Disease. Fat is usually built up in the liver due to obesity, diabetes, or pre-diabetes. Because of America's rise in metabolic syndromes and obesity, many doctors believe these are why the fatty liver disease is also on the rise.

Alcohol-Related Fatty Liver Disease or ALD

ALD, or alcohol-related fatty liver disease, is caused by the heavy consumption of alcohol over time. ALD symptoms include pain in the liver and belly or an enlarged liver. The symptoms and effects of the alcohol-related fatty liver disease will usually get better over time if the person discontinues drinking alcohol. If that person keeps drinking, ALD can lead to alcoholic hepatitis or alcoholic cirrhosis. Alcoholic cirrhosis of the liver can ultimately lead to liver failure, which can lead to death. ALD can comprise of alcoholic cirrhosis, acute alcoholic hepatitis, and simple hepatic steatosis. Having all these illnesses at once is feasible.

When someone abstains from alcohol, the liver will usually go back to regular. Despite the excellent prognosis for alcohol steatosis in the short-term, when patients were followed after treatment, it was found that those with changes to their lives because of alcohol abuse in the past were more likely to develop cirrhosis than others with normal liver function. Doctors use continued alcohol abuse, gender, and extreme steatosis to predict the risk factors of the patient to develop cirrhosis and fibrosis. Females have a higher risk than males.

When the liver has been severely damaged for an extended period of time, most medical professionals considered the outcome of alcoholic cirrhosis is irreversible. Studies are now being conducted that indicate some outcomes, such as cirrhosis and fibrosis, can be reversed depending on the cause and the patient. For example, the patients studied with decompensated alcoholic cirrhosis who got a liver transplant experienced outcomes similar to other liver transplant patients. Their five-year survival rate was about 70%.

The manifest symptoms of alcoholic hepatitis vary because of the disease's wide range in severity. Vomit, nausea, abdomen distention and pain, weight loss, and anorexia are mild, nonspecific symptoms. Encephalopathy, fever, spider angioma, ascites, jaundice, hepatic failure, and hepatology are more specific and severe symptoms. Encephalopathy, fever, spider angioma, ascites, jaundice, and hepatomegaly are noticeable physical symptoms.

Alcoholic hepatitis or fatty liver disease does not always precede established alcoholic cirrhosis. It can begin decompensation without the presence of either. Additionally, acute alcoholic hepatitis may be diagnosed with alcoholic cirrhosis. Other causes of cirrhosis cannot be differentiated from the signs and symptoms of alcoholic cirrhosis. Some of the symptoms and signs of patients include:

- Portal hypertension complications; for example, hepatic encephalopathy, ascites, and variceal bleeding.
- Unusual lab results; for example, coagulopathy, hypoalbuminemia, and thrombocytopenia.
- Pruritus
- Jaundice

A patient who is being evaluated for unusual liver functions test results, such as elevated aminotransferase levels, is the most common diagnostic method for fatty liver disease. There is no specific test available for the fatty liver disease. Most often it is diagnosed when a patient's aminotransferase levels are more than double the normal limits and the results from an ultrasonography. Typically, the findings of an ultrasonography reveal a liver with hyperechoic and may or may not have hepatomegaly.

MRIs or magnetic resonance imaging, and CT scans or computed technology scans are used to diagnose cirrhosis. When reviewing the results of the MRI, unique characteristics can potentially be present with alcohol-related liver disease. For example, it is noticeable if a patient's liver has a larger caudate lobe, the hepatic notch on the right side is more obvious, or the regenerative nodules are larger. It is not typically necessary to conduct a liver biopsy to diagnose fatty liver disease; however, it may be requested to determine fibrosis or steatohepatitis is not present.

Necrosis and inflammation of the liver are the most common and recognizable symptoms of alcoholic hepatitis. These features are the most noticeable in the hepatic acinus' centrilobular region. Reversible portal hypertension and sinusoid compression occur when the hepatocytes become typically distended. Inflammatory cells permeate mononuclear cells and polymorphonuclear cells. These inflammatory cells are typically situated near the necrotic hepatocytes and in the sinusoids. Mallory bodies and fatty infiltration are also often present in patients with alcoholic hepatitis. Mallory bodies are aggregations of the intracellular perinuclear, which is hematoxylin-eosin staining by eosinophilic intermediate filaments. These results are additional indicators of alcoholic hepatitis, but are not required to diagnose the disease nor are particular to the illness.

For patients that abuse alcohol significantly, medical professionals look for the traditional signs associated with the final stage of liver disease to diagnose alcoholic cirrhosis. It is likely that these patients will not accurately share their alcohol consumption, thereby making conversations with friends and family important in estimating the amount of alcohol typically consumed by the patient.

Portal hypertension complications, like hepatic encephalopathy, variceal bleeding, and ascites, can be present in patients with alcoholic cirrhosis. There are no clear findings in pathology that distinguish the advanced liver disease was caused by alcohol or from several other causes. This is especially true when the patient is in the final stage of alcoholic cirrhosis but does not have acute alcoholic hepatitis.

The combination of clinical acumen, laboratory values, and physical findings are an accurate method for clinically diagnosing alcoholic liver disease. A biopsy of the liver is not always necessary, but it can be acceptable in some cases. Typically, when it is uncertain if this is the correct diagnosis, a medical professional will require a biopsy. It is likely that more than 30% of patients are inaccurately clinically suspected of alcoholic hepatitis. Performing a biopsy can confirm the diagnosis. In addition, a biopsy can assist in making decisions on liver therapy, offer a prognosis, determine the amount of damage present, and also rule out additional unanticipated liver disease causes.

Non-Alcoholic Fatty Liver Disease or NAFLD

The non-alcoholic fatty liver disease has a few different forms and serves as a broad-based term for a range of liver conditions. Simple fatty liver disease indicates that the liver has high levels of stored up fat, but may not come with any damage to this liver or inflammation. The simple fatty liver usually will not get worse and doesn't cause any major health issues pertaining to the liver and is the most common type in people with NAFLD.

Non-alcoholic steatohepatitis, or commonly called NASH, is an additional type. NASH means the liver will have inflammation and possible damage to the liver cells. Both the inflammation and cell damage can lead to serious health problems such as liver cancer, cirrhosis, and scarring of the liver and liver failure. NASH is a much less common type of NAFLD but heavy use of alcohol causes damage that is comparable to the damage of NASH.

The common presence of non-alcoholic fatty liver disease is common in the Western nations, but it is spread throughout the globe. In fact, the non-alcoholic fatty liver disease is the most usual chronic liver disease in the U.S. today. It mainly affects people in their 40s and 50s who have type two diabetes or may be at a greater risk of heart disease. Metabolic syndrome, including increased belly fat, high blood pressure and triglycerides, and the body's ability to use insulin, are closely linked to the non-alcoholic fatty liver disease.

A non-alcoholic fatty liver disease may be symptomless at first, or forever. When symptoms of the disease are present, they can comprise liver enlargement, extreme feeling of tiredness or discomfort in the right side of the abdominal area near the liver.

Signs of non-alcoholic steatohepatitis and cirrhosis include large blood vessels beneath the skin, and swelling in the spleen or abdomen, skin, and eyes that begin to turn a yellow color, reddening of the palms and growth of breasts in men. With these symptoms present, making an appointment with a doctor is crucial.

It is unclear to experts why some patients develop a build-up of fat in the liver and others do not develop this illness. In addition, experts are unsure why some cases involve inflammation, which leads eventually to cirrhosis, and other cases do not. The following common links between non-alcoholic steatohepatitis and non-alcoholic fatty liver disease are:

1. Patients who are obese or overweight
2. Patients with a resistance to insulin. Resistance to insulin means your cells do not absorb sugar because of how it responds to the hormone called insulin.
3. Patients with hyperglycemia, or high blood sugar. Patients presenting with this symptom have type 2 diabetes or are pre-diabetic.
4. The patient's blood has high levels of triglycerides or increased fat levels.

A combination of these different issues a patient could present with can lead to the fat build up in the liver. Occasionally, some patients develop fibrosis, or their liver's scar tissues build up because their liver becomes inflamed and non-alcoholic steatohepatitis occurs.

This happens when the patient's body reacts to the increased fat levels as a toxin.

Risk Factors

There are many conditions and illnesses that can raise your risk of developing the non-alcoholic fatty liver disease. Some of these risk factors include:

- Hypothyroidism or a thyroid that is underactive
- Hypopituitarism or a pituitary gland that is underactive
- Type 2 diabetes
- Sleep disorders such as sleep apnea
- Polycystic ovary syndrome
- Abdominal fat concentrations in obese patients
- Metabolic syndrome
- Elevated blood fat, especially triglycerides
- High cholesterol

People most at risk for developing non-alcoholic steatohepatitis include:

- The elderly
- Patients with diabetes including type 1 and type 2
- Abdominal fat concentration in a patient of any weight, however, it is more likely in overweight and obese patients.

Additional testing is necessary to tell the difference between non-alcoholic steatohepatitis and non-alcoholic fatty liver disease. The tests most often used include aspartate transaminase and elevated alanine transaminase. Additionally, many experts will use imaging studies to assist them in diagnosing a patient with non-alcoholic fatty liver disease. Ultrasonography and tomography are two of the more frequently used imaging types when diagnosing nonalcoholic fatty liver disease, however, neither of the procedures can distinguish steatosis and steatohepatitis.

Experts are in controversy over the use of a liver biopsy to diagnose non-alcoholic fatty liver disease. Medical professionals who argue that a liver biopsy is unnecessary cites the following reasons:

1. Risks associated with a biopsy.
2. Few conventional therapies that are available and effective.
3. The disease is generally benign.

There are few risks associated with conducting a liver biopsy, but as many as 30% of patients report transient pain, nearly 3% of patients report severe pain. Less than 3% of patients who undergo a liver biopsy experience substantial complications. Despite the controversy over conducting a routine biopsy, it is generally recommended that patients with advanced liver disease should get a biopsy.

In addition, patients that make significant lifestyle changes but still have continually elevated liver enzymes should be considered for a liver biopsy. The patient should be included in the decision to conduct a liver biopsy and it is recommended by the American Gastroenterological Association to base the decision to conduct a biopsy on each individual case and that the timing should be appropriate for the care of the patient.

Liver Cancer

Cirrhosis is the primary complication of both non-alcoholic steatohepatitis and non-alcoholic fatty liver disease. Cirrhosis is fibrosis or advanced-stage scarring, in the liver. Injury to your liver, like non-alcoholic steatohepatitis inflammation, causes the liver to respond in the form of cirrhosis. Fibrosis or scar tissue is developed by the liver to combat and lessen the inflammation it is experiencing. As inflammation persists, scar tissues continue to build in the liver. Cirrhosis that remains untreated can develop:

- Final-stage failure of the liver. This means that liver ceases all function.
- Liver cancer.
- Hepatic encephalopathy or speech becomes slurred and the patient becomes drowsy and confused.
- Esophageal varices or the veins in the esophagus become swollen. This can result in ruptured veins and internal bleeding.
- Ascites or abdominal fluid buildup.

Patients diagnosed with non-alcoholic steatohepatitis have a 20% chance of progression to cirrhosis.

In the United States, one of the primary causes of hepatocellular carcinoma is NAFLD or non-alcoholic fatty liver disease. Between 2004 and 2009, hepatocellular carcinoma in patients with fatty liver disease rose 5% every year. In addition, patients with fatty liver disease have shorter survival times than those without and when they are diagnosed, the tumor is often more advanced than those who develop this cancer without fatty liver disease. Because of the advanced complications of the fatty liver disease, hepatocellular carcinoma liver transplant is less common.

In a study conducted over a span of five years, liver cancer patients with fatty liver disease were often diagnosed at an older age, were typically Caucasian, and had advanced tumors. Their survival rate for fatty liver disease-related liver cancer was also four months less than those without the fatty liver disease. The study conducted on these patients is extremely significant due to the substantial amount of participants.

Cirrhosis is an indication of liver cancer, but not always, especially if the patient has the fatty liver disease. That is what makes it so challenging to detect and why the mortality rates are poor. A patient that has the fatty liver disease and is obese will typically be monitored more frequently than patients within a normal weight that have the fatty liver disease, primarily because the combination of the two diseases can be a higher risk.

Chapter 2: How the Liver Functions and Types of Liver Disease

Only vertebrae have a liver. No matter the vertebra that has a liver, its role is similar. Specific metabolites are detoxed from the body, proteins are synthesized, and digestion is aided by the production of biochemicals. In humans, it also is responsible for regulating the storage of glycogen, decomposing red blood cells, and producing various hormones.

Located over the intestines, right-hand kidney, and stomach and under the diaphragm is your liver. It takes up the right section of your abdomen's cavity. There are several functions this deep red-brown organ fulfills. Blood enters the liver from two primary avenues: the hepatic portal vein delivers blood rich in nutrients, and the hepatic artery delivers blood filled with oxygen.

The double lobes of the liver each have their own eight sections. Within each various section, there are about one thousand lobules. The common hepatic duct is made up of large ducts that splinter into smaller ducts with connected lobules on the ends. The function of the common hepatic duct is to move the liver cell's bile to the beginning portion of the small intestine called the duodenum, and the gallbladder. Hepatocytes are primarily contained in the liver's tissue. These regulate a large number of reactions of high-volume biochemical. These reactions include complex and small molecules being synthesized and broken down. Many of these reactions are paramount to the body's vital functions.

The liver expels the bile it produces, but the liver also monitors the blood and adjusts the chemical content as needed. Bile is critical in breaking down the fat in order for the body to be able to absorb and digest the necessary nutrients. The liver monitors all the blood that passes through from the intestines and stomach. When the blood enters the liver, the liver determines any imbalance and adjusts it as needed as well as passes on nutrients necessary to healthy bodily function.

Many medications are designed to be broken down and dispersed through the liver. The liver is effective at delivering the medication into the blood in the easiest way for the body to process it. The liver provides some of the most vital functions for the body. The following list contains a short list of the most recognizable functions of the liver:

1. Holds on to and disperses glucose when the body needs it.
2. Delivers fat to the body by producing unique proteins and cholesterol.
3. Develops specific proteins necessary for the plasma in blood.
4. Assists the digestive process beginning in the small intestine by breaking apart fats and removing waste due to the production of bile.
5. Holds on to iron to assist in processing hemoglobin.
6. Urea ammonia, which is harmful to your body, is converted into waste. Urine removes the end-product of the metabolism of protein, urea.
7. Cleanses the blood from harmful toxins like drugs.
8. Ensures that any blood clotting is regulated.
9. Eliminates bloodstream bacteria and develops immune factors to assist the body in resisting various infections.
10. Helps the body remove bilirubin stores. If the body holds on to too much bilirubin, the eyes and skin turn a yellowish hue.

The bloodstream or bile ferries harmful toxins out of your body after the liver has broken them down. Feces leave the body from the intestine, which is filled with the by-products of bile produced by the liver. If a by-product of the bile is filtered through the kidneys first, it leaves the body in the form of urine.

The liver is a gland that assists in digestions because if creates this bile. The bile created is what the body uses to break down fat and is an alkaline compound. When the fat is broken down, lipids remain. Bile emulsifies the lipids, which is how it helps digestion. For many years the function of the organ directly below the liver, the gallbladder, had an unknown necessary function. However, continued research shows that the gallbladder helps the liver by storing bile. No one is certain to this day how many functions the liver undertakes in a humans lifetime, but some texts estimate it has about 500 different roles.

If the liver ceases to function properly, there are a few options for treatment. Over the long term, it is unknown how it is best to make up for the loss of function in the liver. Short-term liver dialysis appears to be beneficial but it is not a long-term solution. There are no artificial livers that have been developed to replace or support a failing or failed liver. The only feasible long-term solution at this time for a failed liver is a liver transplant.

What Are the Different Types of Liver Disease?

The cause of the specific problem is what is used to classify the various types of liver disease. Hepatitis, or liver inflammation, leads to most of the various liver diseases. Hepatitis ranges from life-threatening and chronic to not serious and acute. Other times the issue is an associated part that impacts the function of the liver, for example, the bile duct. This means the disease or issue does not lie in the liver itself but can cause the liver to stop functioning correctly.

Viral Infections

Viral infections are one of the most typical developments of liver disease. These infections inflame the liver, and it is mainly due to hepatitis. Viral infections are classified as A, B, C, D, or E based on the various strains. Hepatitis B is a viral infection transmitted by blood or sexual contact. Hepatitis A is transmitted by food.

Parasitic Liver Infections

Over time the liver can also be damaged by parasites that infect the liver. Liver flukes or blood flukes, different types of flatworms or trematodes, are the most common parasitic liver infection. Snails, cattle, and sheep are the most common carriers for these worms. Humans contract these worms when they ingest food or water that has eggs or immature worms in it.

Alcoholic Liver Disease

Drinking alcohol over extended periods of time is another cause of liver disease. Excessive alcohol consumption leads to damage and inflammation of the liver. A patient with this disease typically has abused alcohol for a length of time and leads to liver failure. Sometimes this disease can be caught in its early stages and can be slowed down when alcohol consumption is stopped. Hepatitis from alcohol is toxic hepatitis.

Alcohol is not the only cause of toxic hepatitis. Several other chemicals can damage and inflame the liver. Some of these chemicals include over-the-counter and prescription drugs, herbal and nutritional supplements, and industrial chemicals like herbicides and cleaning supplies.

Autoimmune Repercussions

When your boy begins attacking itself, it is known as autoimmune hepatitis or autoimmune liver disease. Sometimes it is unknown as to why the immune system attacks the liver and the body, while other times it can be traced back to a source. For example, there are certain genes that can cause this to occur. After a prolonged attack by the immune system, the liver finally becomes inflamed and damaged. Primary sclerosing cholangitis and primary biliary cirrhosis are examples of autoimmune diseases that can cause this form of liver disease.

Genetic Disorders

Genes and genetic disorders are often inherited and lead to various forms of liver disease. Families often experience generational issues with their liver function. Some of these genetic liver diseases include Wilson's disease, hyperoxaluria, and hemochromatosis. Different substances build in the liver when a patient suffers from one of these types of diseases. Copper builds in the liver in patients with Wilson's disease, for example.

Growths, Tumors, and Cancer

The liver can also have a variety of growths and tumors as well as cancer. The growths can be both non-cancerous and benign or can be cancerous or malignant. Hepatocytes, the cells in the liver, cause a liver cancer called hepatocellular cancer. A benign tumor is sometimes a liver adenoma. Another benign tumor is a liver abscess. A liver abscess causes pus to build in the tissue of the liver. Cancer in the bile duct can prevent the liver from functioning properly, but it can also spread to the liver.

Cirrhosis

When the liver becomes scarred and the tissue is destroyed, it is called cirrhosis. This is the final stage of liver disease. Long periods of liver disease or alcoholic hepatitis are two of the most common reasons for cirrhosis to occur. When this occurs, it cannot be reversed. Cirrhosis will lead to death eventually.

Pediatric Liver Conditions

In infants and children, the liver can present symptoms but typically only if it is severely damaged. This is because the liver can regenerate and its reserve capacity is large, especially in children. Some of the liver diseases that are common in children include benign tumors, hepatic hemangioma, Langerhans-cell histiocytosis, alagille syndrome, progressive familial intrahepatic cholestasis, biliary atresia, and alpha-1 antitrypsin deficiency. Benign tumors are considered to be congenital and are the predominant form of liver tumors in children.

A polycystic liver disease is another disorder that begins at gestation and builds throughout the patient's life. It is a genetic disease, meaning, it runs in the family line. This disorder causes several cysts to appear in the tissue of the liver. These cysts typically appear later on in life. They are also typically asymptomatic. All these diseases, including those listed above, can lead to the derangement of the liver's process.

Signals of Liver Issues

The degree and symptoms experienced with liver disease vary from person to person and disease to disease. Despite this, the resulting action on the liver produces common signs even if there are no other symptoms. This is especially true when the disease is in an early stage.

Jaundice or Yellowed Eyes and Skin

One of the most common signals that there is something wrong with the liver is the discoloration of the eyes and skin. A patient suffering from a liver disease will often have a yellow tint in the whites of their eyes and throughout their skin. The yellowing skin color and eye discoloration are called jaundice. When the blood breaks down, red blood cells creates bilirubin that the body needs to excrete. This is usually removed through bile. When the liver is not functioning correctly, it does not excrete this thereby causing the discoloration because the bilirubin begins to build throughout the body. In addition to the yellow color, the skin may become itchy.

Dark Urine And/Or Pale Stool

In addition the yellowing of the skin and eyes, stool and urine may become discolored. Bile leaves the body usually through stool and some through urine, which is how bilirubin is normally excreted. The bilirubin and bile are why stool is a brown color. When the liver is not functioning and bilirubin is building in the body, it is not being excreted through the stool or urine. When this happens, stool color becomes paler. The kidneys begin compensating for the excess bilirubin and try to flush it out more through the urine. This makes the color of urine darker.

Pain in the Liver

The intensity and nature of pain in the liver can vary, and it does not occur in every liver disease. Pain in the liver is located below the right ribcage, in the top right-hand side of the abdomen. Most people's livers sit in this location in their body. A small part of the liver does extend over the middle of the body into the left upper part of the abdomen, so it is possible to also feel pain here, but it is uncommon.

Easy to Bruise

Another signal that there is something wrong with the liver is being able to bruise easily. This symptom can be related to a variety of issues, so it is not isolated directly with liver disease; however, it can indicate something is wrong with the liver. This is especially likely if easy bruising happens alongside any of the other symptoms listed above. Blood clotting is controlled in part by the liver when it is functioning properly. When it is not, the liver could potentially be unable to create enough proteins to clot the blood and prevent bruising. This is why bruising can occur easily, even if the injury was the only minor.

Additional Signals to Watch out For:
- Extreme tiredness or fatigue.
- Abdomen swelling with excess fluid or ascites.
- Additional swelling with excess fluid not in the abdomen.
- No or little appetite.
- Episodes of vomiting or nausea.

Liver Disease Diagnosis

Tests are typically run on a patient when liver disease is suspected. These tests typically include blood tests. These tests look for specific markers. For instance, inflammation or injury appears in the response of the liver by the production of acute-phase reactants.

Chapter 3: What Is a Liver Detox?

Before you embark on a liver detox, it is important that you are aware of the variety of forms a detox can take and also the associated precautions. Liver flushes cleanse or detoxes, terms typically used interchangeably, are a method of supporting your liver remove toxins. Some programs even claim it can purge gallstones!

Prior to beginning any liver detox program, make sure to review what symptoms could occur, what signs you need to be aware of that could indicate an adverse reaction, and what could lead to potentially harmful situations.

There are many detoxes or flushes you can choose from and this variety opens the door for some plans to be labeled as safe and effective when in reality it is harmful and ineffective. Be aware of what choices are available and use your best judgment before beginning any new dietary or lifestyle plan.

The Most Common Liver Detoxes

1. Master Cleanse, AKA the Lemonade Diet

    A diet focused on minor starvation, participants only drink a special lemon drink for ten days while supplementing with laxatives and salt water to assist in defecation. Starvation diets are popular for a variety of reasons but unfortunately, they do worse things for your body than good. They slow down your metabolism and can cause other health concerns like dehydration and disrupted microorganisms. Using laxatives can lower electrolytes and interfere with bowel movements. Laxatives can also interrupt the normal microorganism activity, disrupting digestive functions. Another potentially deadly side effect of this diet, especially when used repeatedly, is elevated acid in the blood, called metabolic acidosis. This diet can disrupt the balance of alkaline and acid in the body, causing severe health complications. Another complication is the production of gallstones. Finally, the overuse of laxatives can create damage to the gastrointestinal tract and develop a dependency on laxatives for elimination.

2. Colon Irrigation, AKA Colonic

   Like an enema, this flush involves flowing water through a tube that is inserted in the rectum to flush out the colon. The purpose is to help remove toxin build up in the colon. The problems with this type of flush are the uncomfortable side effects. For example, vomiting, nausea, bloating, and cramping are all reported, even when an experienced professional do the procedure. Dehydration is another common side effect. More serious health concerns include perforated bowel, colon or bowel infections, and dangerously altered electrolyte levels.

3. Gallbladder or Liver Flush

   Randolph Stone is credited with this detox. Stone instructed his participants to mainly eat apples and drink apple juice. They were to only eat fruits and vegetables and drink herbal tea and olive oil. In addition, they were supposed to inject a laxative, typically water with Epsom salt. This form of a detox is dangerous because it is a form of fasting and also overuses laxatives. Both practices can be very dangerous to your health. In addition, targeting the liver in such a way can potentially release a gallstone from the gallbladder. For people who have gallstones, many are unaware of them until they become lodged in the duct of the gallbladder. When this occurs, it is very painful and emergency surgery is required.

4. Eat Liver-Cleansing Food, AKA the Detox Diet

Some foods are loaded with additional toxins that can "bog down" the liver. For example, foods like sugar, chemicals, fat, and alcohol, can all burden the liver. On this diet, these types of foods should be avoided. Instead, participants focus on foods that support the liver, like apples, walnuts, artichoke, dandelion, grapefruit, and lemon. This is a safe approach to detox, especially when it is paired with an appropriate intake of calories, carbohydrates, and protein.

5. Herbal Supplements for Detox

Many nutraceuticals are available to assist in liver detox. For example, turmeric, vitamin C, N-acetyl-cysteine, alpha R-lipoic acid, and milk thistle have all been shown to support the liver. At the cellular level, the various supplements assist with the detox. In addition, they can protect against damage. It is possible to have a sensitivity or allergy to the various herbal supplements. Before taking anything new, make sure to read and adhere to the instructions. Also, be aware of any reaction or adverse effect it may cause.

Common Detox Symptoms

In addition to the symptoms outlined above, the following symptoms are common while engaging in a liver detox:

- Influenza or the common cold
- Congestion in the sinus cavity
- Trouble sleeping
- Aching body

- Bad-smelling feces
- Diarrhea
- Cough
- Mental fog or confusion
- Irritable
- Anxious
- Dizzy spells
- Acne
- Skin reactions
- Intense or different body odor
- Extreme tiredness or fatigue

Most of the time, these symptoms are an indication that your body is removing toxins from the fat cells throughout the bloodstream. If the symptoms are not severe, they will normally subside once the body has removed all the toxins.

It is typical for some people to react differently to cleansing than other people. Prior to starting a liver detox, make sure to consult your healthcare professional. Seek a physician's support and guidance, especially if you have one or more of the following conditions:

- Chronic liver or kidney disease.
- **Problems with the colon, including colon cancer, Crohn's disease, diverticulitis, or Irritable Bowel Syndrome.**
- Seniors or children.
- Breastfeeding or pregnant women.
- Cardiac disease.
- Hypoglycemia.
- Diabetes.

The Best Detox Solution for You

The most beneficial detox, flush, or cleanse that you could do to support and heal your liver is to eat the best foods and rink the best beverages to aid and ease your liver. This means having a focus on nutritional foods including adequate amounts of water. It is important to avoid fasting or starvation diets including the use of laxatives. These are not beneficial to your body including your liver. If you choose to include an herbal supplement, make sure you choose a reputable brand and source to help protect and support your liver.

It is not simple to detox the liver, and sometimes it is not a pleasant process. But the outcome can be crucial to your longevity and overall health. Despite the many options available for a liver detox, there are some that are not as safe as others. Prior to dedicating yourself to a strict regime, make sure you look into the plan thoroughly and keep an eye out for any negative side effects you are experiencing. This is especially important if you suffer from a chronic illness. If you suffer from something like this, make sure you also work closely with your healthcare providers so you can participate in a gentle and healthy method that is best and most effective for you.

Chapter 4: The Benefits of a Liver Detox

It is common to disregard liver detoxes, but there are several benefits attached to this practice. It spurs healthy eating and also helps you lose unwanted or unneeded weight. Below are some of the most common benefits of a liver detox:

1. Lose unwanted and unneeded weight.

    Fat is broken down in the digestive system by bile, which is produced in the liver. If weight loss is your goal, starting with a liver detox could be a good starting point because this process promotes the production of bile.

2. Support the immune system.

    To have a strong immune system, your liver needs to be healthy. This is because one of the many roles of the liver is to lower toxins in your body. A liver detox can result in boosting your immune system.

3. The risk of liver stones is minimized.

    Excessive levels of cholesterol in the diet can lead to the development of liver stones. Bile hardens when there is excess cholesterol and this hardened bile turns into small stones. These small stones can then restrict the function of the gallbladder and liver. In some cases, you can have as many as 300 liver stones preventing your liver's function! During a liver detox, it is possible and likely to remove 100 to 300 liver stones from your body.

4. A whole body detox is supported.

   Toxins always exist at some level in your liver because of its role in the body's function. It is designed to eliminate toxins by converting them into a byproduct that is harmless to your body. A healthy level of toxins is normal and typically does not create a problem in your body. The problems begin to occur when the toxins build up. To make sure your liver is functioning the way it should, you need to detox your liver.

5. Energy is increased.

   After the liver breaks down toxins into a harmless byproduct, some of the byproducts are used in the body as a nutrient. However, if the liver is blocked with problems like liver stones or toxin build up, these key nutrients never make it to your blood. When your blood does not get the nutrients it needs, you can experience fatigue. To help increase your energy, detox your liver. In addition to experiencing the boost in energy, you will also know that your body is getting the nutrients it was missing before.

6. Vitality improves.

   To return to your ideal proficiency, a liver detox is necessary. Your skin will appear healthier and brighter when you reduce your toxins that have built up in your liver. Your body will respond better to exercise when you support bile production. Some patients and participants feel and appear to be five years younger when they complete a liver detox!

Chapter 5: How to Detox Your Liver Through Diet

The accessibility of fast food, which is often unhealthy and quick, makes any diet or lifestyle change difficult. In order to make changes in your diet, you need to restrain yourself and hold yourself accountable. If you can do this, you can experience life-changing benefits in many areas of your overall health. To detox your liver through diet, consider the following tips:

Tip 1: Eliminate or Minimize Foods That Are Toxic to Your Body

Some foods work against your liver health such as processed foods when your diet includes many of these foods frequently. Processed foods contain ingredients like refined sugar and hydrogenated oils. Foods like processed lunchmeats and convenience foods are known for their toxicity and harmful effects on your body. Hydrogenated oils, or trans fats, contain increased levels of saturated fat. The oil's chemical structure has been engineered to improve the life of the product it is added to. A diet rich in trans fats increases the likelihood of cardiac disease by over 25%. Additionally, it is theorized that trans fats lead to inflammation in the body because it interferes with your immune system.

Other serious health conditions are linked to foods like lunchmeats, fast foods, and convenience foods, which commonly contain added nitrites and nitrates. The purpose of these additives is to retain color in the foods, prohibit the growth of bacteria, and increase the shelf life of the product. Instead of consuming these types of foods, you need to replace them with healthier options that support your liver function. It sometimes requires a little creativity to make healthier options to mimic and replace these unhealthy foods, but you can develop meals that you and your family find full of flavor and supports your liver.

For example, instead of purchasing processed lunchmeats, slice your own roasted turkey or chicken. Homemade granola bars, mixed nuts, carrot sticks, celery sticks, and fresh fruit are all good options to replace a bag or a handful of chips. Instead of making a box of mac and cheese, find a recipe for a healthy alternative such as cheesy spaghetti squash. Potassium, pantothenic acid, manganese, B vitamins, and niacin are all present in spaghetti squash. In addition, spaghetti squash is low in saturated fat and calories. You can add a garnish of crushed walnuts on top to provide a punch of antioxidants and omega-3 fatty acids to also support your heart health.

When you eat foods that are processed, in addition to changing your diet, you also need to ensure that your digestive enzymes properly function. When your liver enzymes are not balanced, you can develop liver and digestion illnesses like Crohn's disease.

Tip #2: Juice Made from Raw Vegetables Is an Effective Delivery Method of Nutrients

A liver detox requires a large number of raw vegetables in your diet, but increasing to the required servings can be impossible for some people. To assist you in getting the vegetable servings you need in an easy way is to juice raw vegetables. One glass of fresh, raw vegetable juice can deliver as much as five servings of raw vegetables that you need. In addition, if you do not like eating raw vegetables, juice can be a tastier and easier way to get the nutrients you require.

Another benefit of raw vegetable juice is that it is easier for your liver to digest. It also makes the nutrients in the vegetables easier for your body to absorb. Some of the most beneficial vegetables in liver detox include Brussels sprouts, cauliflower, and cabbage. The flavors of these vegetables may not sound appetizing; however, you can include other raw vegetables to alter the flavor. Vegetables that are good to add for additional nutrients and flavor include leafy greens, beets, cucumbers, and carrots. All these vegetables assist in developing a balanced pH level by lowering the levels of acid in the body.

Finding a flavor combination you prefer will take some experimentation. Consider adding other fresh, raw juices or fresh herbs to develop a unique flavor. Some flavorful herbs include mint and parsley. One of the most beneficial raw vegetable juices to your liver detox is from organic carrots. Beta-carotene, a nutrient that converts to Vitamin A, is found in carrots. Vitamin A is essential for flushing toxins out of your body as well as reduces liver fat. Ginger root is another beneficial additive to raw vegetable juice. Ginger supports digestion and is anti-inflammatory. Oranges also add a great, sweet and/or tangy flavor to juice. Additionally, oranges deliver Vitamin B6, Vitamin A, and Vitamin C.

Vegetable juice contains a large amount of fiber. High amounts of fiber support your digestion and speed up your elimination process. Having speedy elimination of toxins means your body does not have time to store these, which can build up and harm you.

Tip #3: Foods Rich in Potassium Are Essential

You need to eat over 4,500 milligrams of potassium every day. Are you positive you are getting this recommendation consistently?

Probably not! Foods that contain higher levels of potassium help you lower your cholesterol, support your heart's health, supports your liver cleanse, and reduces your systolic blood pressure. There are potassium supplements available, but you should try to obtain your potassium recommendation through healthy foods such as sweet potatoes, tomato sauces, greens, beans, bananas, and molasses.

Sweet Potato

Many people immediately think that they need to eat more bananas to increase their potassium intake; however, sweet potatoes are actually the richest source of potassium. In addition to beta-carotene and a high amount of fiber, one medium-sized sweet potato delivers about 700 milligrams of potassium. Sweet potatoes are also low-calorie but contain high levels of iron, magnesium, and the vitamins B6, C, and D. Sweet potatoes also have a naturally sweet flavor from natural sugars. The natural sugars are dispersed slowly through the bloodstream thanks to the function of the liver. The beauty of this natural process is that it regulates itself, preventing blood sugar spikes that refined sugars cause.

Tomato Sauce

Tomatoes also contain several nutrients including potassium. When tomatoes are delivered as a paste, puree, or sauce, the benefits of tomatoes are more significantly concentrated. For instance, a cup of fresh tomatoes offers about 400 milligrams of potassium, but a cup of pureed tomatoes contains over 1,000 milligrams! To make sure you get the most benefits in a paste, puree, or sauce, select organic tomato products.

If you intend to make your own concentrate, consider the following recipe to get the most from your effort and the fruit's nutrients:

Ingredients:

- Organic tomatoes, halved

Directions:

1. Warm your oven to 425 degrees Fahrenheit. Place the halved tomatoes on a baking sheet face down.
2. Roast the tomatoes until the skin begins to shrivel.
3. Remove the pan from the oven and allow the tomatoes to cool.
4. Once cool, pinch or slide off the skins and place flesh into a blender or food processor. Pulse tomatoes to gently crush.
5. Pour the crushed, roasted tomatoes into a sieve or strainer to remove seeds, if you prefer. Strain as often you prefer or need.
6. Pour the strained mixture into a Dutch oven or large stock pot on your stovetop. Simmer the sauce for up to 2 hours or until the sauce is thick. Remember, the sauce will continue to thicken after you remove it from the heat, so cease simmering just before the sauce reaches the consistency you prefer.

Leafy Greens

One cup of spinach or beet greens contains a large number of antioxidants and more than 1,300 milligrams of potassium. These ingredients are easy to add to raw juice and can powerfully support the liver. To add these to your diet, chop the vegetables and add to your juice mixture or sprinkle on top of salads. You can also sauté quickly on your stovetop. Additionally, beet greens help the flow of your bile and cleanse the gallbladder naturally.

Beans

There are multiple healthy beans you can choose from to add to your diet. Beans contain a large amount of potassium in addition to fiber and protein. Beans like lima beans, kidney beans, and white beans are all great options and good alternatives to other beans, such as garbanzo beans. Instead of making hummus from garbanzo beans, try one of the other beans in your recipe and enjoy your new creation with celery sticks and carrot sticks.

Molasses

Just any molasses is not the best source of potassium; however, blackstrap molasses can provide a significant portion of your recommended daily value of potassium in addition to other nutrients like copper, manganese, calcium, and iron. In fact, just 2 teaspoons of blackstrap molasses provide about ten percent of the recommended amount of potassium.

An easy way to incorporate blackstrap molasses into your diet is by replacing other sweeteners you use. Use it in porridge made with quinoa, on top of steel-cut oatmeal, or make homemade BBQ sauce with it. Even stirring the two teaspoons into your morning coffee is an excellent way to add sweetness as well as nutrients. The added benefit of adding blackstrap molasses to your coffee is that it enriches the flavor while reducing the acidic taste.

Banana

Bananas are rich in potassium. Adding a single medium banana to a smoothie is a great way to increase your potassium and sweeten the drink. A medium banana delivers about 470 milligrams of potassium, digestion support, and release of heavy metals and toxins from your body. When you are going through your liver detox, these benefits are essential. Make sure you always have enough bananas on hand to add to your foods or to snack on during your detox.

Tip #4: Do an Enema with Coffee

An enema assists with constipation, but an enema with coffee also helps you regain more energy and support your liver detox. Enemas target the bottom part of the large intestine. There are many ways and resources to help you complete it at home, unlike other interventions, like a colonic. Colonics target the full bowel and requires the assistance of a professional. This makes an enema a more accessible and "attractive" action to assist in your liver detox. You can purchase an enema kit at most drug or convenience stores.

When doing a coffee enema, organic coffee is kept in your bowel. By retaining it in your lower part of the large intestine, it allows the wall of the intestine to absorb the coffee liquid and transport it to the liver. The absorption of the organic coffee stimulates the production and flow of bile. This stimulation kick starts your liver and gallbladder. When your liver and gallbladder are kick-started, you begin to produce glutathione, a chemical compound that is a strong cleaner. This chemical compound aids in the elimination of the toxic build up in your body.

Moving out toxins quickly is essential during your liver detox. To give yourself a coffee enema, boil three cups of distilled or filtered water with 2 tablespoons of ground, organic coffee. Once the mixture reaches a boil, lower the heat and simmer for about 15 minutes. When done, let the mixture cool to room temperature. Once the coffee mixture is completely cool, strain it through a cheesecloth to remove all the sediment from the liquid. Use this liquid in your enema kit. Once the liquid is inserted, aim to keep the liquid in for up to 15 minutes. When you reach 15 minutes or your limit, release.

Tip #5: Supplements for Turmeric, Dandelion, and Milk Thistle Are Beneficial

Turmeric

Various health conditions, such as chronic pain, prostate health, breast health, osteoarthritis, depression, cancer, and Alzheimer's disease, are all subjects of current scientific research being conducted on the effect of turmeric on these conditions. Preliminary results already show that turmeric can support liver metabolism and tissue, regulates the balance of our blood sugar, assists digestions, minimizes pain in the joints, and helps minimize depression. More benefits are expected to emerge as research is continually published.

Dandelion

Many people who have to maintain any sort of lawn hates dandelions. This weed moves freely and infests the ground every spring and throughout the summer. While it may be a nuisance in the yard, these little flowers contain beneficial minerals and vitamins from its pedals to its roots. When you ingest dandelion, you help your liver detox easier by acting as a diuretic and speeding up toxin elimination. Additionally, dandelion helps upset digestion, heartburn, unbalanced blood sugar levels, and a weakened immune system. You can take dandelion root as a supplement or drink it in an herbal tea for your liver detox.

Milk Thistle

An ideal detox herb is milk thistle. Many familiar with this herb consider it the "king" of herbs used for detox. This is why it is so important and valuable during your liver detox. Part of the benefit of consuming milk thistle includes removal of alcohol in the liver, pollutants from the environment, prescription medicines, and heavy metal build up. For patients undergoing radiation or chemotherapy, they experience a series of unwelcome side effects, which milk thistle can help reduce. To support the regeneration of the liver, the silymarin active in milk thistle is beneficial to the strength of the liver's cellular walls. Take a milk thistle supplement or drink it in an herbal tea designed for your liver detox.

Bonus! Burdock Root

Similar to dandelion, this root is helpful with detoxing your blood, which then aids the function of the liver. Similar to milk thistle, burdock root can also be taken as a supplement or in a liver detox tea.

Tip #6: Take Liver Supplements or Eat Organic Liver Meat Regularly

Consuming organic liver meat from young and healthy chicken or cattle that is grass-fed contains the most coQ10, chromium, zinc, copper, iron, choline, and folic acid, vitamin A, and B vitamins. The get the most nutrients from a food, you cannot do better than eating liver.

If eating liver is not an option, ingest beef liver supplements. Make sure to choose supplements that offer a guarantee that no antibiotics, pesticides, or hormones are used in the care and feed of the animals. This ensures you get the best and most nutrients in the supplements.

Chapter 6: Natural Remedies for Fatty Liver Disease

Currently, there are only two primary therapies offered for NAFLD. The first is using medications and pharmaceutical interventions. The second is intervening in your lifestyle. Intervention includes engaging in or increasing physical exercise, modifying your diet, or reducing your body weight. The most common therapy is lifestyle intervention, specific modifications to your diet and reducing your body weight. These two often go hand-in-hand. Metabolic diseases, such as hyperlipidemia and obesity, as well as NAFLD, can be slowed through moderate and long-term exercise.

Despite the knowledge that intervention in your lifestyle can reduce the progression of NAFLD, the mechanisms underlying this benefit are still unknown. Several published scientific studies illustrate the benefits of lifestyle intervention, but none firmly put a finger on the reason for it. Still, it is undeniable the potential for therapeutic benefits. These natural interventions, or remedies, have more beneficial outcomes in scientific studies than pharmaceutical interventions. Pharmaceutical therapy includes various drugs, including renin-angiotensin system blockers, lipid-lowering agents, insulin sensitizers, and antioxidants. Some studies on animals and cells show promising results, but few clinical trials on humans are positive.

There are several beneficial effects in herbal remedies for NAFLD cessation. Attention to these natural remedies has increased in recent years because they are available around the world; typically have little or no side effects, and multiple clinical and basic studies support their effectiveness.

Current Natural Remedy Findings for Treating NAFLD

Goji Berry, Wolfberry, or Lycii Fructus

From the Solanaceae family, goji berry is the fruit from the Lycium Barbarum. Chinese medicine made this fruit famous for its benefits on the eyes and liver. The LBP, or the polysaccharide part of the fruit, is the most beneficial part of the goji berry. Results of modern studies show that LBP has a variety of benefits biologically, including a reduction in the risk tumors, maintenance of glucose metabolism, neuroprotection, immunoregulation, and antioxidant abilities.

Additional clinical studies show that the juice of LBP increases the amount of immunoglobulin G, levels of interleukin-2, and lymphocytes in humans. Reducing the formation of lipid peroxide and increasing antioxidant serum levels are additional benefits of LBP.

Early findings show that LBP prevented propagation and encouraged hepatoma cells apoptosis in the liver. An additional study illustrated LBP's protective attributes when incorporated in a diet high in fat that caused oxidative stress injury in the liver. In these situations, LBP increased the activity of antioxidant enzymes and the products of oxidative stress to help protect against further oxidative stress injury in the body. Other studies showed the powerful healing properties of LBP in alcohol-related fatty liver disease and how it can aid in the regeneration of the liver.

Garlic or Allium Sativum

There is a long history of medicinal and culinary uses of garlic in the Mediterranean region, Egypt, and Asia. A recent report published that eating a whole piece of garlic helped improve blood glucose resistance, lipid metabolism, and oxidative stress. Reduced activity of the cytochrome P450 system and increased antioxidant activity resulted in one study when black, aged garlic was combined with the administration of chronic ethanol in rats. Garlic has also been found to help protect and repair liver damage from CCl4. When paired with other medicinal and natural remedies, garlic enhances the beneficial effects of reducing steatosis, inflammation, oxidative stress, and fibrosis. Finally, garlic also helps prevent further damage to the liver for patients with NAFLD.

Green Tea

Another natural remedy is the green tea plant. This remedy is one of the most documented plants used to prevent liver problems. In the last two decades, increased attention on the beneficial and healing properties of this plant has supported its capabilities in liver health. The plant Camellia Sinensis provides the leaves used in making green tea. The plant was originally found in China but it spread across Asia to places like Vietnam, Korea, and Japan. It has now spread to Western locations, infiltrating into black-tea cultures.

Mice treated with CCl4 were also given pure EGCG, or epigallocatechin-3-gallate, in one impactful study. EGCG is green tea's primary polyphenol. The result showed benefits on a biochemical and histological level. It impacted inflammation, oxidative stress, and helped resolve liver injury. In another recent study, EGCG was shown to prevent the entrance and passage of hepatitis C. Obese lab rats in a study conducted on liver disease and EGCG found benefits on both the health of the liver and the reduction of unwanted weight.

Resveratrol

Red grapes contain a phytoalexin that can be extracted, which is called resveratrol. It is well documented to protect against inflammation and oxidative stress. It is one of the most accepted natural remedies because of its powerful properties and its worldwide availability. Recent studies have shown that resveratrol is an effective treatment for NAFLD. This is an effective remedy to use every day to prevent and heal fatty liver disease.

Milk Thistle

As mentioned in the previous chapter, milk thistle is a beneficial plant during a liver detox. Milk thistle is in the daisy family and produces two important derivatives, silymarin, and silybin. There have been more than 10,000 reports published over the past ten years on the benefits of milk thistle on the body, and specifically liver health. The findings in these reports link the effects of the two derivatives to hepatoprotective, chemopreventive, and antioxidant results. In the liver specifically, silymarin and silybin improve the effects of antioxidants. They also, directly and indirectly, impact fibrosis and inflammation in the liver. An additional study shows that patients suffering from chronic hepatitis C and NAFLD, they experienced better effects of silymarin because of the increased concentrations of flavonolignan plasma and wide-ranging enterohepatic circulation.

Additional Decoctions and Derivatives to Consider

Additional natural remedies that have been used in traditional Chinese medicine and are now supported through experimental biology, pharmacology, and chemistry, include berberine. The herb Coptidis Rhizoma from China contains this isolated alkaloid, which has an anti-steatotic effect. It also reduces the inflammation response from hepatitis. Currently, there are no modern studies directly linking berberine to the treatment of NAFLD.

Additional Natural Suggestions

- Minimize sugar intake to less than 30 grams per day.
- Reduce stress.
- Slow down your pace of living.
- Place a castor oil pack over the liver a few times a week.
- A couple times a week eat organic organ meats.
- First thing in the morning drinks eight ounces of beet kvass.
- Incorporate low-impact and stress-relieving physical activity such as yoga or walking into your weekly activity.

Chapter 7: Healthy Diet Foods and Drinks for Fatty Liver Disease

Almost one-third of the adult American population is affected by fatty liver disease. It is on the primary causes of liver failure and once the liver fails, there is no long-term treatment option other than a liver transplant. Many cases of the fatty liver disease are not diagnosed until late in the disease, making some of the damage irreversible. However, it is possible to prevent and treat the disease to improve your length and quality of life. One of the most common methods of prevention and treatment includes dietary changes. It does not matter if you have an alcoholic fatty liver disease or non-alcoholic fatty liver disease, diet can improve your liver's health.

The general rules to follow for a liver-healthy diet includes:

- Do not consume alcohol.
- Consume a very small amount of saturated fats, refined carbs, trans fats, salt, and sugar.
- Modify your diet to include several whole grains and plants that are high in fiber, such as legumes.
- Eat large amounts of vegetables and fruits.

Because the fatty liver disease is a build-up of fat in the liver, reducing the additional fat you intake is important. You can also focus on reducing your caloric intake to aid in weight loss, which can also help relieve fatty liver disease and additional stress on your body. When you lose unwanted weight, you lower the risk of contracting the fatty liver disease. If you are overweight, set the goal to lose about 10% of your current body weight.

How to Heal Fatty Liver Disease Through Food

Listed below are some of the best foods and drinks you should consume during a liver detox and while supporting your healthy liver function.

1. **Coffee**

    You are welcome, coffee lovers! Reports have shown that drinking coffee helps reduce unusual enzymes in the liver. In addition, patients with fatty liver disease that also drink coffee regularly often have less damage to their liver than those that do not drink it. Moderate amounts of caffeine can minimize abnormal liver enzymes, which is especially important for people who are at risk of developing the fatty liver disease.

2. **Leafy greens**

    These superfoods also block the buildup of fat. For example, broccoli prevented fat build up in the liver in rats in one study. Spinach, kale, and Brussels sprouts also aid in weight loss. Look for recipes that use a lot of leafy greens to get a powerful punch every day.

3. **Tofu**

    Tofu is a good source of protein and is also low fat, but it is the soy protein in the food that specifically benefits those suffering from fatty liver disease. Rats in a study at the University of Illinois revealed the power of tofu and soy protein in protecting against the fat build up in the liver.

4. **Fish**

   Lower inflammation and improve the fat levels in the liver with the support of omega-3 fatty acids. These beneficial acids can be found in foods like trout, tuna, sardines, and salmon. These are all considered "fatty" fish but they provide a healthy fat that your body can break down easily versus other fats that are easily stored in the liver. When preparing fish, remember to focus on keeping the recipe low-fat because the fish already contain enough fat for your body.

5. **Oatmeal**

   When you are struggling with fatigue as a side effect of fatty liver disease or during the early stages of treatment for the disease, it can be hard to function properly. Eating whole grain carbohydrates like oatmeal can provide your body with a boost of energy that can sustain for long periods of time. In addition, the fibers in oatmeal help make you feel full and sustain that feeling of fullness. Finally, oatmeal has also been shown to assist you in maintaining a healthy body weight.

6. **Walnuts**

   Another food high in omega 3s is walnuts. When patients with fatty liver disease consume a small handful of walnuts, often they have better liver test results.

7. **Avocado**

   Protect your liver by eating healthy fats like those in avocados. Current research shows that avocados contain specific chemicals that potentially reduce damage to the liver. Avocadoes are also a rich fiber source, which also aids in losing weight.

8. **Low-fat dairy and milk**

   A study published in 2011 on rats reported that whey protein in milk can help protect against liver damage, even if damage already exists. Consume a glass of milk per day or about eight ounces of organic, grass-fed animal cheese for optimal results.

9. **Sunflower seeds**

   Vitamin E is high in sunflower seeds and is known for its antioxidant properties. Antioxidants help your liver protect itself from further damage.

10. **Olive oil**

    A third source of omega 3s on this list. Choose this oil instead of butter, shortening, or margarine while cooking. Olive oil has also been shown to control healthy weight levels and reduce the level of liver enzymes.

11. **Garlic**

    As mentioned earlier in this book, garlic is helpful in protecting and supporting the liver as well as promoting healthy body weight. It is also very flavorful so it can make many dishes delicious quickly. It is a good source for burning built up and unwanted fat in the body.

12. **Green tea**

    Another repeat food on our list, green tea has been shown to help you absorb and process fats in the body, rather than storing them in your liver. It has also been linked with improved liver function. Other benefits include sleep assistance and reduced cholesterol.

Additional Liver-Supporting Foods

- Beets
  Rich in antioxidants and activates liver enzymes, also improves bile production and improves physical activity.
- Organic apples
  Rich in fiber, especially with the skin on, and make sure the fruit is organic because apples tend to be one of the top fruits and vegetables to have excessive amounts of pesticides on them.
- Broccoli sprouts
  Strong detoxifier, rich in antioxidants, boosts glutathione more than just broccoli, contains a hormone regulator called indole-3-carbinol, and contains cancer-fighter sulforaphane.
- Fermented foods such as sauerkraut, kefir, kombucha, kimchi, or pickles. Promotes digestion and elimination through good bacteria compounds.
- Citrus fruits such as lemons, limes, oranges, or grapefruit.
  Helps the liver cleanse and create enzymes for detox.
- Carrots
  Rich in beta-carotene and plant-flavonoids, and contain Vitamin A for liver disease prevention.
- Most forms of vegetables.
  Cauliflower and broccoli contain glucosinolate for detoxing enzyme production and sulfur for overall health in the liver. Spinach and other leafy greens are rich sources of chlorophyll to assist in removing toxins from the blood and also provide an alkaline balance to the heavy metals in the liver.

Additional Liver-Supporting Beverages

- Blueberry juice: Fibrosis, which is the scarring that is the result of liver disease, was the topic of the study published in the journal PLOS One on March 2013. The animals in the study were fed blueberry juice to observe the effects it has on fibrosis over a period of eight weeks. The results of the study indicate that blueberry juice has the ability to both increases the liver's capacity to stand levels of oxidative stress and increase proteins that support the liver to fight against fibrosis. Oxidative stress occurs when cells are damaged by free radicals which are unstable molecules.
- Blood orange juice: In 2012, a study published in the World Journal of Gastroenterology concluded that fat accumulation is prevented when participants regularly consumed blood orange juice. Over the span of 12 weeks, the obese animals in the study were fed the juice every day. According to the study, the rats experienced several healthy responses, including improved insulin sensitivity, reduced triglycerides, and overall cholesterol, lowered body weight, as well as provide protection against fat build up in the liver. The hormone, insulin, regulates blood sugar levels. It is important that the body is sensitive to this hormone so it can regulate blood sugar appropriately. If the body does not have a stable sensitivity to the insulin, it is possible and likely the person will develop diabetes.
- Noni fruit juice: Noni is a plant that grows in tropical climates and bears noni fruit. It is botanically known as Morinda Citrifolia. Health stores are the primary vendors for noni

juice supplements in the United States. It is likely that you will find noni juice mixed with other fruit juices, most commonly grape juice. The conclusion from the 2008 study on animals that was published in the journal Plant Foods and Human Nutrition shows damage from toxins in the liver is minimized when the participants drank noni juice regularly.

- A note on fruit juice: Fruit juices often contain added refined sugar. Make sure to read the labels carefully. Choose juices that have no or little sugar added and also look for the juice content. Try to purchase juices that are labeled as 100% juice, if possible. Many juice brands will include only a small portion of fruit juice in their bottle. This often occurs with blueberry juice. Juice also contains high caloric levels and the fiber from the fruit has been removed. You will get far less fiber than if you were to eat the whole fruit by itself. For those interested in juicing your fruit, keep in mind that some fruit is only available seasonally. For example, blood oranges are in stores from the month of January through the middle of April. If you can find them in stores outside of those times, they will most likely be more expensive and not great quality.

Avoid the Following Foods:

1. Salt: Too much salt makes your body retain water. Make sure not to consume more than 1,500 milligrams per day.
2. Red meat: These culprits are sources of unwanted saturated fats. Beef and deli meats specifically should be avoided.
3. White pasta, rice, and bread: White foods indicate that it has been processed. Processed foods raise your blood sugar and lack fiber and other nutrients that their whole grain counterparts offer.
4. Fried foods: Anything fried will be high in calories and unhealthy fats.

5. Additional sugar: Fruit juices, sodas, cookies, and candy are all high in refined and added sugar. These raise your blood sugar and can increase fat build up in your liver.

An Example Diet Plan

The next chapter will cover meal plans and recipes in more depth, but provided below is a sample meal plan to illustrate what a fatty liver diet and detox can look like.

Meal Time	Breakfast	Lunch	Dinner	Snacks

Menu	8 ounces of coffee with skim or low-fat milk 1 cup of whole-grain oatmeal topped with 2 tablespoons almond butter and 1 medium banana, sliced	8 ounces low-fat milk 1 medium apple 8 ounces steamed broccoli, carrot, or other leafy green 1 small baked potato 3 ounces grilled chicken 1 cup fresh spinach topped with olive oil and balsamic vinegar	8 ounces steamed broccoli, carrots, or another vegetable 8 ounces mixed fresh berries 8 ounces of low-fat milk 1 whole-grain roll 3 ounces of baked salmon a small mixed-bean salad	2 teaspoons of hummus with fresh vegetable sticks OR 1 tablespoon almond butter spread over sliced fresh apples

Additional Natural Remedies Suggestions for Fatty Liver Disease

Other natural remedies to consider do not include diet. These changes can improve your overall health, including your liver function. Some of these remedies include:

- Increasing your physical activity.

When you pair a diet with exercise, you not only lose the excess and unwanted weight, but you also can manage your general health and liver disease with this combination. The goal should be a minimum of 30 minutes of moderate to high-activity several days a week.

- Reduce your cholesterol.

If you are not able to lower your cholesterol through diet and exercise alone, you may need to work with your healthcare professional to begin certain medications to assist you. It is important to lower your triglyceride and cholesterol levels. You can do this through your diet by minimizing or eliminating added sugar and saturated fats.

- Keep diabetes in check.

The fatty liver disease often accompanies diabetes and vice versa. Changing your diet and your physical activity levels are effective treatment methods for these two diseases. If these two remedies do not drop your blood sugar levels to a healthy level, you should speak with your healthcare professional to stabilize your blood sugar with medication as well.

Chapter 8: Eating Plans and What Foods and Drinks to Avoid

Have you decided that this is the weekend you are doing a liver detox or cleansing? If you are still on the fence about the idea, maybe you should put it on your agenda. A detox has the reputation of being a life-disrupting and challenging undertaking, but a short detox focused on healthy foods is easier and less painful than you are probably imagining. Your liver is an incredibly important organ in your body, and your skin is the only larger organ you have. A detox is a way you can help it function better every day by giving it a break from foods that are hard to process, that are filled with preservatives and are toxic to your health. Your liver supports most of your bodily functions including your digestion, reproduction, immunity, and hormones. Even your skin is supported by your liver function.

It can do all of this work because of the nutrition it derives from what you eat. Juice diets are a common detox method used to help your body remove toxins, but they are challenging to stick to. Dietitians and nutritionists are now more likely to suggest and support a food-based cleanse. A detox that focuses on foods that provide your liver with the "right" nutrients makes it easier for participants to stick to, especially if they are new to detoxing. It is far easier and less of a commitment than doing a traditional juice cleanse. In addition, during a juice cleanse, participants often struggle with metabolic slowdown and withdrawal and deprivation feelings. Doing a food-based detox; however, minimizes these side effects.

Foods to Avoid in Your Liver Detox Eating Plan

The great news is that you can eat during your detox! You get to eat a lot of great foods and counting calories is not really the focus of the plan. Instead, you are focused on increasing the "good" while minimizing or eliminating the "bad." Below is a list of the few types of foods you need to avoid while participating in your cleansing:

1. Soy products, except for tempeh if you typically consume soy products.
2. Corn
3. Red meats or other fatty meats. If you eat meat regularly stick to lean, roasted chicken breast.
4. Canola and vegetable oils.
5. Coffee
6. Alcohol
7. Condiments like ketchup and mayonnaise.
8. Foods high in sodium or added salt.
9. Processed or fried foods.
10. Gluten products like pasta and bread.
11. All dairy products.
12. Foods high in sugar especially added refined sugar. Fruit and its natural sugar are ok in moderation during the detox.

Tips on How to Get the Most from Your Liver Detox Eating Plan

Before you whip up recipes and plan out your weekend of meals, consider the eight tips below before you get started so you can get the most out of your time.

1. Plan on drinking eight ounces of water with a fresh lemon wedge the first thing in the morning. This helps get your

body hydrated and ready to flush out the stagnant toxins from overnight.

2. Drink half your body weight in water every day. Consider adding a teaspoon of chlorophyll or spirulina powder to eight ounces of water to boost your detox. You can add this to your water up to three times a day during your detox.
3. Choose organic foods whenever you can to help cut out added hormones and toxins.
4. Sprinkle flax or chia seeds on your foods. These contain a rich dose of fiber, which helps your colon remove the toxic waste from your liver. You can also create a flax tea by steeping 1 tablespoon of flax in eight ounces of hot water, then straining the liquid to remove the seeds before drinking.
5. Stock up on foods that are liver-healthy such as cilantro, parsley, watercress, spinach, cucumber, radish, broccoli, asparagus, lime, lemon, and apple. These can be easily eaten on the go or added to other foods for additional flavor and benefits.
6. Plan to make a green smoothie or juice every day. The liquid state helps your body digest the nutrients and also allows your liver to absorb what it needs for optimal health. Consider adding a cup of spinach or leafy greens to a handful of other fruits and vegetables for a lunch alternative or afternoon "snack."
7. Two hours before bedtime, you should stop eating. Your liver works through the night to remove toxins from your body while you sleep so do not give it an overload right before it starts its hardest work.
8. Allow yourself to get all the rest you need. Sleep helps your body reset and restore, so make sure you give it the time while you detox. When you focus on resting, your body can

promote the ideal function of all your organs, including your liver, and support your digestion.

Eating Plan Menu and Detox Plan Sample

Friday Evening

Begin by going to the grocery store and purchasing the fresh foods you need for this weekend. Eat a filling, healthy dinner with a lot of vegetables and about three ounces of a lean protein, preferably fish like salmon or tuna. Before you go to bed, prepare a chia seed pudding with a handful of fresh fruit on top for an easy morning meal tomorrow. As you settle into bed, drink eight ounces of filtered water with a fresh lemon wedge or a cup of turmeric tea. Make sure you go to bed early enough so you can get eight hours of good sleep.

Saturday Early Morning

First thing, when you wake up, drink eight ounces of filtered water with a fresh lemon wedge or a cup of unsweetened green tea. Eat your chia seed pudding, and add seeds or nuts to the top, if you prefer. Walnuts, pistachios, sunflower seeds, or pumpkin seeds are all good options. These nuts or seeds will help add fiber to the meal and also help you stay fuller for longer.

Saturday Late Morning

If you are beginning to feel hungry but it is too early for lunch, prepare a green smoothie or fresh green juice. Make sure to include a leafy green with fruits and vegetables with no added sweetener. Bananas and unsweetened coconut milk are good options to add a little sweetness naturally.

Saturday Afternoon

For lunch, cook kelp noodles and top with sliced vegetables in a rainbow of colors. Consider orange and purple carrots, beets, bell peppers, etc. If you need protein and more filling foods, roast the tempeh to add in the top of the salad. On the side, slice an organic apple with a dollop of unsweetened almond butter for dipping.

Saturday Late Afternoon

If you begin to feel hungry after lunch but it is too early for dinner, grab a handful of carrot stick or another fresh vegetable. A small handful of walnuts, cashews, or almonds are another good afternoon snack. Sip on lemon water throughout the day, especially if you are feeling hungry but you have just eaten something. Your body is most likely thirsty, not hungry if this is what you are feeling after a meal or snack.

Saturday Night

Prepare a healthy meal full of vegetables and seeds. Consider adding fresh vegetables to a large butter lettuce leaf spread with unsweetened almond butter and sprinkled on top with sunflower seeds. Enjoy a glass of organic or homemade kombucha. Before going to bed, place a castor oil pack over your liver and then treat yourself to a warm Epsom salt bath. Head to bed at a good time to make sure you get your full eight hours of sleep.

Sunday Early Morning

Pour yourself a bowl of gluten and grain-free muesli mixed with unsweetened almond or coconut milk. Top it with fresh fruit and seeds, if you prefer. Sip on a cup of green tea or mix fresh blueberries, a lemon wedge, and cucumber slices into eight to ten ounces of filtered water to drink.

Sunday Afternoon

Spiral cut a zucchini to make a "zoodles" and toss with a fresh pesto made with herbs, olive oil, crushed walnuts, and garlic. Serve with a bowl of cool avocado soup.

Sunday Late Afternoon

For a snack, enjoy a sliced apple or radish or prepare a homemade hummus with liver-healthy beans and serve it with sliced vegetables. Fill your afternoon with light activity such as meditation or yoga or a short, leisurely walk. Make sure to drink plenty of filtered water flavored with lemon or cucumber.

Sunday Night

Top a large, leafy green salad with 1/3 cup tempeh, roasted chicken, or beans and a balsamic vinegar and olive oil dressing. In your blender, add one cup of spinach with blueberries, pineapple, and a banana to make a tasty green smoothie to drink. Before bed, place another castor oil pack over your liver and take another Epsom salt bath, if you would like. Make sure you go to bed at a decent time so you can get your full eight hours of sleep again.

Monday Morning Through Night

Continue a modified detox breakfast so you do not shock your body with old, unhealthy foods. Instead, enjoy ½ avocado sliced on top of scrambled eggs or another chia seed pudding with nuts, seeds, and fresh fruit. Drink eight ounces of water with a lemon wedge or a cup of green tea before any coffee. Try to continue eating many fruits and vegetables throughout the day and do not drink any alcohol tonight.

A 24-Hour Liver Detox

If you are not interested or able to do a weekend detox, consider doing a 24-hour cleanse. The week leading up to the day of your cleansing, make sure you eat a lot of the following foods:

- Celery
- Beets
- Asparagus
- Citrus fruit
- Brussels sprouts
- Broccoli
- Cauliflower
- Lettuce
- Cabbage
- Kale

Avoid alcohol and processed foods leading up to the day of your cleanse as well. On the day of your cleansing, make 72 ounces of the following liquid to drink throughout the day. Also, make sure to drink at least 72 ounces of water.

24-Hour Detox Drink

Ingredients:

- Cranberry juice
- Nutmeg
- Ginger root
- Cinnamon
- Fresh orange juice from 3 oranges

- 3 Lemons

Directions:

1. In a large container, mix three parts water to one part cranberry juice.
2. In a large saucepan, steep ¼ teaspoon grated ginger root, ¼ teaspoon nutmeg, and ½ teaspoon cinnamon in four cups of water. Simmer for 20 minutes.
3. Let cinnamon, ginger and nutmeg liquid cool to room temperature.
4. Juice the oranges and lemons into the liquid and stir to combine.
5. Combine the infused liquid with the cranberry juice and stir well.

Easy Detox Soup Recipes
Broccoli Soup

Ingredients:

- Coconut oil, 1 Tsp.
- Broccoli florets, 2 cups
- Celery stalks, chopped, 2
- Parsnip, peeled and chopped, 1
- Garlic cloves, minced, 2
- Carrot, peeled and chopped, 1
- Onion, chopped, 1
- Low sodium vegetable stock, 2 cups
- Spinach, 2 cups

- Lemon, juiced, ½
- Chia seeds, 1 tbsp.
- Sea salt, ½ tsp.
- Mixed nuts and seeds, toasted, if preferred.

Instructions:

1. In a large stockpot, warm the oil over low heat. Combine the broccoli, celery, parsnips, carrots, garlic, and onion and cook for five minutes. Stir often.
2. Pour in the broth and boil. Cover with a lid and lower to a simmer. Simmer for 7 minutes or until vegetables are cooked but not too soft.
3. Mix in the spinach and then pour mixture into a blender. Add the lemon and chia seeds. Blend until creamy.
4. Add salt as preferred and serve with warm, toasted nuts and seeds, if desired.

Beet Soup

Ingredients:
- Beets, medium, cubed, 3
- Coconut oil, 1 Tsp.
- Carrots, diced, 2
- Leek, small, diced, 1
- Garlic cloves, minced, 1
- Onion, diced, 1
- Vegetable stock, warm, 2 cups
- Sea salt, ¼ tsp.
- Chia, pumpkin, and sunflower seeds, if preferred.

Instructions:

1. In a large stockpot, place the beets inside and cover with water. Bring to a boil and then lower the heat. Simmer uncovered for 30 minutes or until the beets are tender.
2. Drain the beets from the water and allow it to cool.
3. In a large skillet, warm the oil over low heat. Combine the carrot, leek, garlic, and onions and cook for seven minutes. Place vegetables on a plate to cool.
4. In the blender, combine the beets, vegetables and warm stock. Blend until smooth.
5. Add salt as preferred and serve with warm, toasted nuts and seeds, if desired.

Conclusion

Thank you for making it through to the end of *Fatty Liver Diet – Guide on How to End Fatty Liver Disease*, let's hope it was informative and able to provide you with all of the tools you need to achieve your goals whatever they may be.

The next step in preventing or healing fatty liver disease is to break out your calendar and decide when you are going to start your liver-healthy diet. If you are unsure about how you will do with making a life-changing diet, start with the 24-hour detox. Pick up a few of the ingredients and choose a day to focus on your liver. If you feel ready for more of a challenge, block out a weekend for the 2½ day diet. Whatever you decide, just make sure you decide to focus on improving your liver function and heal fatty liver disease.

After you figure out when you are going to do your detox, continue to stay focused on your liver health. Continue to boost your health by nourishing your body through healthy meals. Review the liver-supporting foods listed throughout this book and stock your fridge and pantry with things you can integrate and grab when you need to. Make it easier on yourself to always have these foods on hand and a few recipes you can rely on when you are in a pinch. Give the recipes in the last chapter a try, but come up with a few of your own based on your own food preferences.

The diet plan in the last chapter is designed to give you quick and easy options to help you cure fatty liver disease and support your liver healthy. The liver detoxes here are focused on providing your body with the nutrients it needs as well as support the liver's health. As you have learned, this is not a book about how to lose weight while doing an unhealthy (and inefficient) liver detox. This is about supporting your health and liver by curing fatty liver disease. If you struggle with fatty liver disease or another liver issue, it is important that you make the suggested changes to your diet, not just when you are completing a liver detox, but as often as possible. Follow your fatty liver diet and enjoy the benefits of a healthier, happier you.

CPSIA information can be obtained
at www.ICGtesting.com
Printed in the USA
LVHW082347170120
644096LV00012B/306